The Complete Electric Pressure Cooker Cookbook

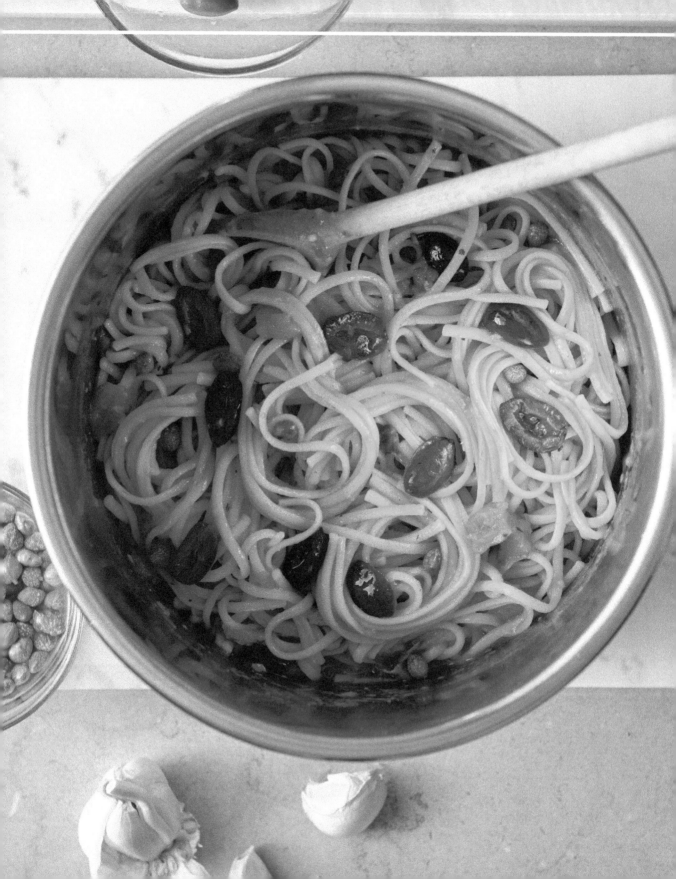

THE COMPLETE
ELECTRIC PRESSURE
COOKER COOKBOOK

150 Simple Recipes Perfect for Any Type of Cooker

Kristen Greazel

PHOTOGRAPHY BY DARREN MUIR

ROCKRIDGE
PRESS

Interior and Cover Designer: Darren Samuel
Art Producer: Hannah Dickerson
Editors: Greg Morabito and Van Van Cleave
Production Editor: Ruth Sakata Corley

Photography © 2020 Darren Muir, food styling by Yolanda Muir

Hardcover ISBN: 978-1-63878-812-6 | Paperback ISBN: 978-1-64739-150-8 | eBook ISBN: 978-1-64739-151-5
R0

For Greg, Evan, Jack, and Will and for the rest of my family.
The year 2020 made me realize how much I cherish our times together.
When this is all over, let's get together as much as we can!

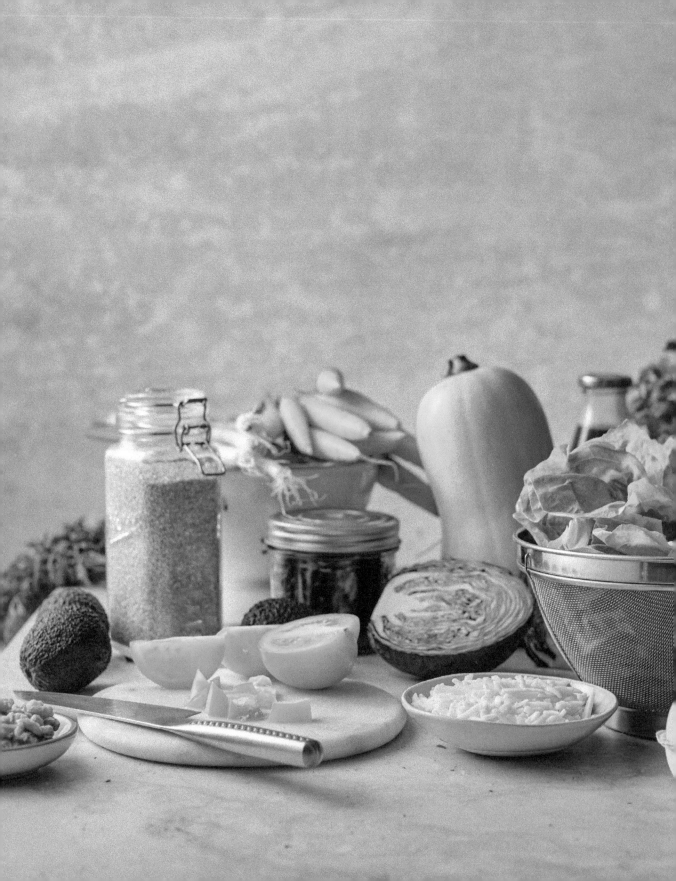

Contents

Introduction

Sitting around the dinner table with family and friends is my favorite place to be. I find serving nourishing meals to my loved ones to be incredibly rewarding, and after I got on board with the electric pressure cooker trend, my love for cooking only grew stronger. When you cook meals in a pressure cooker, you don't need to choose between serving healthy meals and spending time on the other important areas of your life. Families these days are busier than ever. An electric pressure cooker can help relieve a little of that stress around mealtime.

I first heard about pressure cookers when my mom told stories about my great-grandmother, Mary. She raised her children during the Great Depression and made delicious meals in her pressure cooker from leftovers because she didn't believe in letting food go to waste. Mary made amazing chicken dumpling soup out of leftover dinner scraps and often cooked cinnamon applesauce with the apples that grew in her yard.

All these years later, I now prepare many fantastic meals of my own, sometimes using leftovers, in my electric pressure cooker. It is incredible how an electric pressure cooker produces meals that taste as though they slow-cooked all day, even if they took under an hour to make from start to finish. I have a newfound love for many different foods after cooking them in my pressure cooker. In 2016, the first thing I made in my first pressure cooker—I now own three—was pulled pork, and I was so blown away with how terrific it tasted that I haven't cooked pulled pork any other way since!

Besides the convenience and flavor-boosting factors, there are several other benefits to using modern electric pressure cookers. Most have a sauté function, so you can also make other elements of your meals, either before or after the pressure-cooking process. I love cooking entire meals in one pan, which saves my family loads of dishes. And modern electric pressure cookers are versatile: You can prepare foods that fit any diet for any meal of the day.

If you're new to the world of pressure-cooking, figuring out how to start can be overwhelming—but it doesn't have to be. Even if you are a rookie, I am here to help! The recipes in this book will help you gain a better understanding of how to use the various settings, how long to cook different foods, and how to optimize the use of each function. And if you're a seasoned pressure cooker user, you will undoubtedly pick up some new tips and ideas that will inspire you.

I am a busy mom of three young sons living in the Midwest. I like to serve quick, kid-friendly meals that are both nourishing and budget-friendly, ideally using as few dishes as possible. Throughout this book, I will share recipes that taste good enough for company but are easy enough to throw together before soccer practice on a Tuesday. I will also share recipe variations and my favorite ways to use leftovers for delicious lunches and "round two" dinners.

And easy dinners are just the tip of the iceberg. I promise that once you learn to use your electric pressure cooker as a soup maker, slow cooker, vegetable steamer, egg poacher, cake-baking vessel, and homemade yogurt-making machine, you will be hooked!

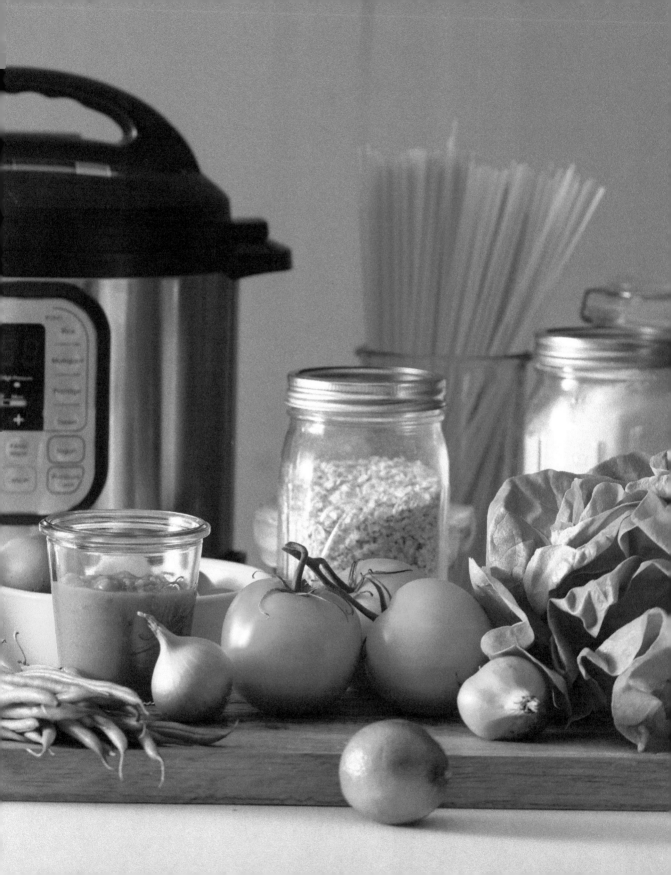

1

The Fundamentals of Electric Pressure Cooking

This chapter will help you understand how to use your electric pressure cooker. In addition to information on when to use the various buttons and pressure release methods, this chapter also includes an overview of some of the more unique uses of this appliance, such as sous vide and canning. Once you are acquainted with your machine, you can start to get creative in the kitchen.

A FASTER, EASIER WAY TO COOK YOUR FAVORITE FOODS

With all of us trying to achieve more with less time nowadays, it's no wonder that electric pressure cookers have become so popular. Making recipes in an electric pressure cooker drastically reduces cooking time and lets you create meals with a hands-off approach. One of the reasons why these devices are so popular is their versatility: Electric pressure cookers allow you to prepare stews, grains, dried beans, and pot roasts, all with minimal fuss. Several cooking functions are possible with this one appliance. You can use it to sauté, cook rice, make yogurt, can fruit or vegetables, braise meat, make sauces and condiments, or create desserts. Once you've learned all of your electric pressure cooker's different functions, it will be super easy to use and will become a permanent presence on your kitchen countertop.

Here are a few advantages to owning an electric pressure cooker:

» **You can achieve perfect-tasting, tender meat in a fraction of the time of a slow cooker.** You can cook large cuts of meat such as pork tenderloins, beef roasts, and hams in under 45 minutes, while those same cuts of meat might take 6 to 8 hours in a slow cooker.

» **You can make homemade pasta dishes with a hands-off approach.** Pasta recipes will require half the cooking time than the time on the pasta box. This allows you to make a pasta dish without standing by the stove, stirring the sauce all afternoon.

» **You can cook dried beans in minutes without soaking them overnight.** Usually, beans need to be soaked overnight, then cooked for several more hours. In the electric pressure cooker, presoaking beans is not necessary.

» **Pressure cooker foods retain more vitamins and flavor than boiled food.** When an ingredient is boiled, its nutrients are lost to the cooking water. However, in a pressure cooker, the liquid stays in the pan—and so do the nutrients!

» **Cooking homemade stock takes way less time.** You can make stocks easily out of your leftovers right after dinner and be able to store them before bedtime. This is much more convenient than making them in a slow cooker or on the stovetop.

» **Delicious pot roasts will cook in a fraction of the time they would take in the oven.** Instead of making large roasts in the oven, heating up your kitchen and requiring to supervise, you can take the hands-free approach by cooking them in the pressure cooker.

The Science of Pressure Cooking

When an electric pressure cooker is set to pressure cook, the cooking liquid's temperature will rise rapidly and create steam. The steam will then build up inside the sealed inner pot and create pressure while the air is expelled out of the appliance. Once the pressure cooker pot is sealed, the hot steam under pressure will cause the food inside the device to cook rapidly. This process is the same for traditional stovetop pressure cookers, but unlike their electric counterparts, stovetop cookers rely on an outside heat source, do not automatically regulate their temperatures, and do not have built-in timers.

Electric pressure cookers are smart machines that control the temperature depending on the cooking method. For example, when using the "soup" button, your device will regulate the heat source to keep the inner pot's contents from getting burnt on the bottom. Most cookers have several other dish-specific buttons that will automatically cook foods at high pressure for different periods of time, plus buttons to use for steaming, sautéing, and slow cooking.

GETTING TO KNOW YOUR POT

Although there are many brands of electric pressure cookers on the market, they all share a standard set of parts and controls. They might seem intimidating at first, but they will become second nature after you start using your cooker.

The Parts

Before you start using your electric pressure cooker, it's important to know about the parts of this appliance, the function of each of its buttons, and some of the key terminology that pops up in recipes.

Control panel: The control panel is on the front of the pressure cooker. It contains all the cooking function buttons and is where you adjust the cooking time and the temperature.

Cooker base: The cooker base is the outside of the electric pressure cooker and contains the control panel.

Float valve: The float valve is a little stainless steel disc in the pressure cooker lid that tells you if the device has come to pressure. When the float valve pops up, the pressure cooker has come to pressure and the cooking time should begin soon after. When you release the pressure, the float valve will pop back down, which indicates that you can safely open the pressure cooker.

Heating element: The heating element is located at the bottom of the pressure cooker and heats the inner pot.

Inner pot: This is the stainless steel pot that comes with your device.

Lid: The lid is vital to the functionality of your electric pressure cooker. You will need to close the lid and lock it securely every time you pressure cook. The float valve and the steam release handle are both on the lid.

Lid position marker: The lid position marker shows you where your lid should be on the pressure cooker so that the lid secures.

Liquid trap: Some electric pressure cooker models come with a liquid trap. It attaches to the pressure cooker base just below the rim and will reduce messes by collecting any liquid before it gets on your countertop.

Sealing ring: The sealing ring is the removable silicone ring in the lid. This ring must be installed properly for your machine to pressurize correctly. You need to wash the sealing ring between uses.

Steam release handle: The steam release handle is also referred to as the "steam release valve." It is used every time you use your cooker for pressure-cooking. The switch can be turned to either "sealing" to secure the pressure or "venting" to release the pressure.

Trivet: The trivet is a metal rack with collapsible sides. It is an excellent accessory for creating many different recipes!

The Controls

The control panel includes several parts that will help you keep track of your cooking process: Mode indicators show you which cooking method has been selected; the pressure indicator indicates whether the cooker is operating at high or low pressure; and the time display shows how many minutes you have chosen to cook, how much time remains in the cooking process, and how many minutes your pot has been naturally releasing pressure. The control panel also includes buttons that will allow you to start and stop the appliance's various cooking methods. These functions are labeled slightly differently from brand to brand, but they all typically operate in similar ways. Here's a guide to the buttons that you will find on most electric pressure cookers:

Manual/Pressure Cook: Most cookers have buttons either labeled "manual" or "pressure cook" that start the pressure-cooking mode. Users can select either high or low pressure, either by hitting "adjust" or the "pressure level" button. (Most of the recipes in this book instruct you to set the pressure cooker on high pressure.) This step is followed by pressing the "+" or "–" buttons to set the cook time outlined in each recipe. Electric pressure cookers can cook anywhere from 0 minutes to up to a few hours. When you set the pressure cooker to cook for 0 minutes, your pot will come to pressure and then turn off the heat source, at which point the pressure will start to come down.

Sauté: The sautéing function saves my family so much kitchen cleanup. I hit the "sauté" button to sauté onions or meat before the pressure-cooking process begins. I also use it at the end of the cook time to thicken soups, stews, and sauces. In most pressure cooker models, you can lower or raise the temperature by either hitting the "adjust" button or pressing the sauté button again.

Slow Cook: If your electric pressure cooker resides on your countertop, there is no need to get your slow cooker out. The slow cooking function on most pressure cookers is very easy to use. Just add the food to the bottom of the inner pot, secure the lid, and hit the "slow cooker" button. You set a cooking time by pressing "+" or "−." You can also adjust the temperature by hitting the "adjust" button, or, in some models, pressing the slow cooker button again. When slow cooking, you will leave the steam release handle at "venting."

Steam: The "steam" function is very easy to use and makes deliciously steamed vegetables and fish. All you need to do is place 1 cup of water into the electric pressure cooker pot, followed by the wire trivet. Place your food on top of the trivet, secure the lid, set the steam release handle to "sealing," and cook. You want to use a quick pressure release when you use the steam function or your food can get overcooked quickly.

Beans/Chili: This automated function is ideal for cooking dried beans without any soaking necessary. The normal setting cooks the beans at high pressure for 30 minutes, but the timing can also be adjusted in either direction if you want beans that are softer or firmer.

Meat/Stew: Use this button for pressure-cooking thick pieces of meat and hearty stews. On most cooker models, this mode will cook the food at high pressure for 35 minutes on the standard setting. The time can also be adjusted depending on the cut and quantity of meat; selecting "more" will increase the cook time to around 45 minutes, while selecting "less" will reduce the cook time to 20 minutes.

Multigrain: Use this setting to cook grains like wild and brown rice at high pressure for approximately 40 minutes on the standard setting, 20 minutes on "less," or 60 minutes on "more." Since the release methods and grain-to-liquid ratio are crucial to using this function, consider consulting the Pressure-Cooking Time Charts (page 237) before you start cooking.

Porridge: The normal setting will cook rice-based porridge (such as congee) for around 20 minutes at high pressure. Adjust to "less" for cooking oatmeal, and "more" if using a mixture of grains and beans.

Poultry: Use this automated feature to cook chicken, turkey, or duck at high pressure. The standard setting will cook the poultry for 15 minutes.

Rice: The "rice" button on electric pressure cookers might be my favorite function. I used to make rice in a traditional rice cooker, and it took forever compared to the 12 minutes it typically takes in the electric pressure cooker. Just add the appropriate rice-to-water ratio to the inner pot, secure the lid, rotate the steam release handle to "sealing," and hit this button. The cooker will automatically adjust the cooking time based on the volume of rice and water in the pot.

Soup: This automated setting cooks the ingredients for 20 to 40 minutes at high pressure, depending on the setting, without the soup boiling too heavily.

Yogurt: Once you start making yogurt in your electric pressure cooker, you will never buy store-bought yogurt again. You hit the "yogurt" button and your electric pressure cooker will cook the milk at 180°F, then the yogurt will begin to culture when it cools down. The cooking process for yogurt takes several hours but is worth the wait.

[−] and [+]: After selecting your cooking method, use these buttons to adjust the cook time.

Keep Warm: Your electric pressure cooker will automatically switch over to "keep warm" when the pressure-cooking process has ended, but you can also disable this mode at any time by hitting this button. "Keep warm" is an excellent function for people who like to make meals a few hours ahead of time or if you want to use the pressure cooker as a serving vessel for a get-together. And if you don't want to further warm or cook the food, simply hit "cancel."

Adjust: This button allows you to set the pressure level (typically low or high) before cooking. On some models, this key is labeled "Pressure Level," while on others, the pressure can be adjusted by simply holding down the "pressure cook" or "manual" button until the desired pressure level is selected.

Delay Start: Some cooker models have a feature that allows users to delay the start of the cooking process. After entering the cooking method and cook time, press this button and use the "−" and "+" buttons to select how long you want to delay the start of the cook time.

Cancel: This is the button that stops the heating process. When using sauté mode, you must hit this button before switching to another setting, such as pressure-cooking or slow cooking. The cancel button will also turn off the "keep warm" setting once you're finished cooking; in some models these functions are combined on a "keep warm/cancel" button.

Once you try a recipe with each button on your electric pressure cooker, you will become familiar with and less overwhelmed by its options. All you need to do is figure out which button to use, set the time, adjust the steam release handle, and determine the method of pressure release and the cooker will do the rest of the work for you.

Pressure Release Methods

As you read the recipes in this book, you'll notice two terms that are distinct to electric pressure cooker usage which will come up over and over again: natural pressure release and quick release. Here's everything you need to know about these two methods:

Natural Pressure Release: When the cooking process is completed, you will hear a beep. Natural Pressure Release means you don't turn the steam release handle but instead let the cooker reduce pressure naturally. A natural pressure release will typically add between 10 and 15 minutes to the overall time, but this can vary depending on how much food and/or liquid is in the pot. When the float valve pops down, the pressure has been released from your cooker and it is safe to open. The setting on the pressure cooker will automatically change to "keep warm" mode once the lid is open (unless you have opted to turn off this function). To turn off the heating unit completely, press "cancel."

Quick Release: A quick release is what happens when you flip the steam handle to "venting" as soon as cooking is complete. It takes about 1 minute for the steam to escape and the pot to fully depressurize. The steam is very hot and can burn you, so please keep your hands away from the steam. Some recipes call for a natural release for a certain number of minutes followed by a quick release (this combination is sometimes called an "abbreviated release"), while other recipes will sometimes call for short intervals of quick release (a process sometimes called "intermittent release"). For simplicity's sake, the recipes in this book will only refer to these two main forms of release—quick or natural—even when they are used together.

Taking It Slow

Did you know that you can also slow cook in your electric pressure cooker? While pressure-cooking might be the most popular mode, most brands of cooker come equipped for slow cooking. Using your device as a slow cooker is a great way to make a meal when you're out of the house all day.

- Many soups and meat dishes can be adjusted for the slow cooker. You can still use the sauté function before you slow cook your meal.

- There are several recipes in this cookbook that can be easily adapted to the slow cooker mode: Shredded Greek Chicken (page 134), Creamy Chicken with Cornmeal Dumplings (page 140), and French Onion Pot Roast (page 188) all taste delicious cooked using the slow cooker mode.

- The one downside for me in using the slow cooker mode is that I like to look through the slow cooker's lid. There are, however, clear glass lids you can purchase for your pressure cooker if you plan to use the slow cooker function often.

HOW TO USE YOUR COOKER

The pressure-cooking process is easy once you get the hang of it. To start things off, place the inner pot into your electric pressure cooker, attach the power cord, and plug it in. The display on the control panel will light up when it is successfully connected. If you're browning or sautéing any ingredients before pressure-cooking, select the "sauté" setting and wait for the pot to heat up for approximately 2 minutes before adding any ingredients.

Once it's time to pressure-cook, place your ingredients in the inner pot and either select a cooking mode like "rice" or "poultry" or select "pressure cook" plus the desired cook time. Secure and lock the lid, set the steam release handle to "sealing," and wait for the device to achieve pressure—this usually takes between 5 and 10 minutes, but it can take longer depending on the amount of food in the pot.

Once the cook time has completed, either let the pressure release naturally by waiting until the float valve has fully dropped (5 to 15 minutes) before unlocking the lid, or opt for a "quick release" by turning the pressure release valve to "venting" and waiting for the pressure to fully release (about 1 minute). When you open the lid, open it with caution, because even if all the pressure has been released, there will still be hot steam that can cause burns. It is essential to read the safety tips in your electric pressure cooker manual before using it.

You will need to clean your electric pressure cooker after each use. The inner pot, sealing ring, float valve, steam release handle, and lid can be washed in the dishwasher or by hand. You will need to remove all the small pieces when you are cleaning these items. Washing the smaller parts in the basket in your dishwasher works well. The detachable power cord, outer pot, and display can be cleaned with a damp cloth. Cleaning the rim on your electric pressure cooker can be tricky. I always twist a cloth to get access to the rim. You can also use a sponge, a Q-tip, or a thin bottle brush to get at the rim's residue.

Some pressure cooker recipes require a sling to remove the food from the inner pot safely. You can either buy a silicone sling or make one out of aluminum foil. An example of a recipe you would need a sling for is a cake. You can create an aluminum foil sling by taking a 20- to 25-inch length of foil and folding it into thirds. You should place the foil sling under the cake pan to lower it into the pot onto a trivet. Then use the ends of the sling to remove the cake pan when it's done.

ELECTRIC PRESSURE COOKER DO'S AND DON'TS

Modern electric pressure cookers are equipped with more safety features than the device my great-grandmother used. However, it is still important to use your pressure cooker correctly. Here are a few do's and don'ts for safely and correctly caring for your machine.

DO'S

» DO place your electric pressure cooker away from your kitchen cabinets. Letting out steam underneath your cabinets can damage the woodwork.

» DO wash the sealing ring in the dishwasher after making aromatic, savory dishes.

» DO use an oven mitt to avoid burns when releasing steam, removing the lid, and removing the inner pot.

» DO use at least 1 cup of liquid when cooking in your electric pressure cooker to avoid burning your food.

» DO remember to place the inner pot in the electric pressure cooker before you start adding ingredients. If you don't, you'll have a big mess on your hands.

» DO make sure that you cover pasta entirely with water. This will avoid burning.

DON'TS

» DON'T overfill the inner pot; overfilling can clog the venting knob and disrupt the cooking process.

» DON'T try to remove the lid when your machine is coming to pressure. This can result in scorching steam and liquid bursting out. Lifting the lid can be very dangerous. If you absolutely need to remove the lid at this point in the cooking process, press cancel and wait a few minutes until the pressure has dropped before venting and removing the lid.

» DON'T use the quick release for soups, stews, or chilis. This can cause your meal to splatter, along with the steam. It can create a big, hot mess.

» DON'T place your hands directly in the steam when it is releasing. The steam is hot and will burn.

» DON'T place a cloth barrier on the steam release handle when your electric pressure cooker is quick releasing, because the cloth will get scalding hot.

» If you own more than one inner pot, DON'T stack them when storing. They can stick together and be hard to separate.

» DON'T place your electric pressure cooker on your stovetop. If your stovetop gets turned on, the heat will melt your machine.

ADDITIONAL COOKING TOOLS AND ACCESSORIES

Your electric pressure cooker is a versatile machine that can cook in so many ways. However, there are a few kitchen tools and accessories that will make the process easier. Here is a list of accessories that will help you get the most out of your electric pressure cooker and prepare the recipes in this book. You probably own many already, and the others on the list are worth the investment.

Must-Haves

Cutting board and knife: These two kitchen staples are absolutely essential for ingredient prep.

Kitchen shears: Use the shears to cut food items right into the pot.

Measuring cups: These ensure that the correct amount of liquid is added to the pressure cooker.

Oven mitts: Always use these to protect your hands from burning when handling the lid or inner pot.

Ramekins: Mini ramekins are used for personal-size omelets and desserts, as well as for canning.

Tongs: Tongs help you remove cuts of meat, potatoes, and other larger items from the pressure cooker's inner pot. It's good to have multiple pairs.

Vegetable steamer: A basic mesh steamer basket is good when using the steam mode on your electric pressure cooker. I use my vegetable steamer for cooking potatoes, vegetables, and fish. There are also times when you need something shallow for when you are stacking ingredients. This can be just be an old-fashioned collapsible metal steamer.

Nice-to-Haves

7-inch springform pan: These are for making cakes or cheesecakes.

Extra inner pot: Having an extra inner pot is incredibly useful when making more than one electric pressure cooker recipe in a day.

Extra sealing rings: You need to wash sealing rings after each use, so extras are convenient. You won't have to wait to use your electric pressure cooker again.

Glass lid: This is good to have when using your electric pressure cooker as a slow cooker.

Silicone molds: These molds with small cups are used for making individual desserts and for cooking eggs.

Silicone sling: If you have this handy tool, you won't have to make a sling from aluminum foil.

BUILDING YOUR PANTRY

Here is a list of items I always have in my pantry. Most of these items should be available at your local supermarket. I also buy a few of the "hard-to-find" ingredients on Amazon.

Grains

- Arborio rice
- Cornmeal
- Farro
- Jasmine rice
- Pasta: thinner and smaller pasta shapes cook best
- Quinoa
- Steel-cut oats

Pantry

- Canned beans
- Canned tomatoes
- Capers
- Chicken stock

- » Cornstarch
- » Dijon mustard
- » Honey
- » Kalamata olives
- » Lemon juice
- » Soy sauce
- » Sugar

Oils

- » Olive oil
- » Sesame oil
- » Vegetable oil

Herbs and Spices

- » Black pepper
- » Chili powder
- » Cinnamon
- » Cumin
- » Dill
- » Garlic (freeze-dried)
- » Ginger
- » Greek seasoning
- » Herbes de Provence
- » Italian seasoning
- » Sage
- » Sea salt

Freezer

- » Bacon
- » Corn
- » Fruit
- » Mixed vegetables
- » Onions, shallots, and celery: Buy fresh in bulk, prep them, and freeze in sealed bags

My Five Favorites

Here are my five favorite recipes from this book:

Tomato Risotto (page 104): In my twenties, I would always look forward to visiting home, where my mom waited with homemade risotto for dinner. I never thought I could make anything close to her creamy, comforting risotto. But making this rice dish in the electric pressure cooker is so easy and delicious! Although it's not my mom's version, this recipe is fantastic, quick, and fancy enough to serve to company.

Chicken, Bacon, and Ranch Casserole (page 142): Learning how to make a "dump and go" casserole was a game changer for cooking healthy, comforting meals for my family in a pinch. You can use either fresh or leftover chicken breasts in this casserole. Both mixed vegetables and leftover veggies from your refrigerator work well. I made this casserole for a quick hot lunch often during the 2020 quarantine, and it felt good to provide my children with the comforts of home during that challenging time.

Turkey Meat Loaf and Mashed Potatoes (page 152): As a child growing up in the Midwest, meat loaf was a regular meal, but I shied away from making it as an adult because of time constraints. Electric pressure cooker meat loaf turns out flavorful every time, and I love cooking this recipe all in one pot for a quick dinner. I have spent years playing around with ingredients to make the perfect meat loaf glaze. Although I always look forward to using leftovers for a meat loaf sandwich the next day, I hardly ever have any.

Large-Batch Smoky Barbecue Pork Chop Sandwiches (page 172): In the Midwest, large family get-togethers, potlucks with friends, and buffet meals happen for almost every occasion imaginable. Every Midwest cook needs a few go-to main dishes to serve a crowd. This recipe fits that bill. It requires only a few easy ingredients, cooks up fast, and is always a crowd-pleaser!

Ground Lamb Shepherd's Pie (page 198): This shepherd's pie filling turns out so flavorful and comforting, and the potatoes are always cooked velvety and smooth. Shepherd's pie is a dish that will please everyone and, in my opinion, is appropriate for any time of the year.

ADAPTING RECIPES

It's fairly easy to convert your family's cherished recipes to work in the electric pressure cooker if you follow a few basic guidelines. Recipes that adapt easily include most slow cooker dishes, soups, stews, chilis, meats, beans, grains, casseroles, and pastas. Here are some tips to keep in mind when adapting these recipes:

» Consult the Pressure-Cooking Time Charts (page 237) to get a sense of how long you should be cooking your dish for and at what pressure level.

» The general rule for pasta dishes is that 1 pound of pasta needs to cook in 4 cups of liquid. The pasta cooking time should be half of the cooking time you see on the pasta box.

» If you cook soup or a stew in the electric pressure cooker, any milk or thickeners, such as cornstarch, should be added after the pressure-cooking is done.

» Most basic rice recipes can be cooked using the "rice" button, and most basic soups using the "soup" button.

» Adding enough liquid is important for adapting a recipe to the electric pressure cooker. At least 1 cup of liquid is needed for the electric pressure cooker to achieve pressure.

Some recipes will not adapt easily, such as fried or crispy foods. Expensive cuts of meats that are best served rare or medium-rare will not be successful. Also, cooking vegetables along with meat may turn the vegetables into mush. A chicken and broccoli recipe, for example, would require adding the broccoli after the pressure-cooking process.

Adjusting to High Altitude

If you happen to live in an area of high altitude, you will need to adjust your cooking time to get the appropriate results, because water evaporates faster at higher altitudes. Most electric pressure cooker manufacturers recommend increasing the cooking time by 5 percent for every 1,000 feet over 2,000 feet of elevation. For example, if you live at 3,000 feet above sea level, multiply the cooking time by 1.05. If you live at 4,000 feet above sea level, you will need to multiply the cooking time by 1.10, and so on.

EASY TRICKS AND TIME-SAVERS

Cooking in an electric pressure cooker will save you time and money and reduce stress. You can cook whole foods like beans, grains, eggs, vegetables, and meats in a fraction of the time. Making home-cooked meals and prepared lunches is an easy way to save money. Packaged food and fast food should become scarce at home when your family can eat nutritious meals from your electric pressure cooker. Here are a few more techniques that will help you save even more time!

Pot-in-Pot

Pot-in-pot cooking, also known as PIP, is an electric pressure cooker technique that many users love. The pot-in-pot technique is used when different foods are cooked in separate pots or sections simultaneously within the inner pot. Here are some tips for the pot-in-pot cooking method:

» A general rule is that meat goes on the bottom of the inner pot, with vegetables on top.

» You will want to use the Pot-in-Pot method with foods that are generally very moist. Vegetables, for example, stand up well to PIP-style cooking.

» Make sure you use ovenproof bowls and pans.

» Never cook a completely frozen dish using this cooking method. It can cause the dish to shatter.

» Add about 5 minutes to the cooking time when cooking meats.

» Look for this method in many of the dessert recipes in chapter 8.

Equipment for pot-in-pot cooking:

7-inch bowls: Ovenproof bowls or baking dishes can be stacked.

7-inch pans: Cake pans can be used to separate elements of a meal.

Aluminum foil: You can wrap elements of a meal in foil if you intend these items to steam. You will want to fold a packet for your food, but don't seal it 100 percent.

Stackable pots: There are stackable pots designed specifically for the pot-in-pot method.

Trivets: The trivet that comes with your electric pressure cooker can separate elements within the inner pot.

Vegetable steamers: A collapsible metal vegetable steamer works well to separate elements within the inner pot.

Parchment paper: You can also wrap different foods in parchment paper packets and cook them in separate areas within the inner pot.

A few recipes in this book that use the pot-in-pot method include Roast Beef Sundaes with Horseradish (page 192) and Ground Lamb Shepherd's Pie (page 198). Both recipes will instruct you to cook the meat in the bottom of the inner pot, with the potatoes on top of the trivet or in a foil packet on top.

Meal Prep

Meal prep has taken off over the last few years as more and more people are trying to eat healthier without spending a lot of time in the kitchen during the week. An electric pressure cooker makes prepping meals ahead of time so much easier. Here are ways you can meal prep with your electric pressure cooker:

» Any meal in the day can be prepped ahead. Breakfast could be Ricotta Egg Bites (page 41); Farro (page 67) makes the basis for lovely lunch bowls; and meats, stews, and casseroles are perfect for dinner.

» What I call "bag and pen" freezer meals save lots of time during the week. This process involves prepping the raw ingredients for a meal ahead of time and freezing. Use a pen to mark the bags with what recipe the ingredients are for (and also the date that you bagged it). When it is time to make a quick meal, remove the frozen bag, thaw it in warm water, toss it into the electric pressure cooker's inner pot, and cook! I like to prepare "bag and pen" meals after returning from the grocery store with a large meat package. Instead of placing that meat in the refrigerator or freezer, I prep it for easy freezer meals.

» When meal prepping in freezer bags, remember to add enough liquid, so you won't need to think about it when you are dumping the freezer bag into your electric pressure cooker during the dinnertime rush.

» I like to menu-plan weekly or bi-weekly. I also like to date my meal prep freezer bags so that I don't forget what's in them.

» A few recipes in this book that can be prepped as "bag and pen" freezer meals include Chimichurri Beef Stew (page 90), Chicken Fajitas (page 139), and Cinnamon Applesauce Pork Chops (page 171).

Cooking Off the Cuff

Once you get acquainted with your electric pressure cooker, you may be inspired to whip up delicious meals with what you've already got in your kitchen. I have created some of my favorite recipes over the years by just making do with what I had available. Once you figure out the order in which the ingredients need to be added to the pot and the cooking methods involved, you can have a lot of fun cooking on the fly.

» Understanding the pressure cooker's sautéing function will help you sauté onions and sear meat for delicious meals. The pressure cooker's sautéing function is also used to thicken soups, stews, and sauces after they've come down from pressure.

» Keep in mind that broths, sauces, and other liquids count as the "liquid" needed for the electric pressure cooker to achieve pressure.

» Remember that vegetables, meats, and onions also contain liquid. You might find that less liquid is needed when using these ingredients.

» Once you understand basic formulas for certain meals, you can adapt them and make them your own—use the recipes in this book as inspiration and consult the Pressure-Cooking Time Charts (page 237) as needed.

BEYOND THE BASICS

Many newer models of electric pressure cooker have two features that are perhaps not for everyday cooking but are definitely worth trying if you're curious: sous vide and canning.

Sous Vide

Sous vide is a cooking method that originated in France that involves cooking food in plastic bags submerged in water that's kept at a controlled temperature. This method is often used in high-end restaurants to cook vegetables and pricey cuts of meat and fish to perfection. All of the flavor is captured inside the bag. Meat turns out almost velvety and vegetables turn out perfectly al dente. Many newer electric pressure cooker models have a sous-vide mode that you can use.

While some chefs spend their whole careers perfecting the art of sous vide, the basic steps are actually fairly simple. To start, place the ingredients that you want to cook in a plastic freezer bag and press out as much air as possible before sealing the top. Fill three-quarters of the inner pot with water, add a trivet or steam rack to the bottom, and place the lid on the cooker without sealing it. Press the sous vide button and use the "–" and "+" controls to adjust the temperature. Press the sous vide button once again and use the "–" and "+" controls to select the cook time. The cooker will beep when the desired temperature has been reached. That's when it's time to place the sealed bag with the ingredients inside the cooker, making sure that the ingredients are submerged while the seal stays above the water. Place the lid back on the cooker and set it to "venting." Once the cook time is complete, remove the bag, take out the ingredients, and check for doneness using a digital thermometer.

Using the sous-vide method, chicken breasts typically take 1 hour at 155°F to be cooked to perfection, while steaks generally need 1 hour 30 minutes at 130°F for medium-rare meat. (See your cooker's manual for more info on sous vide times and temps.) If you want to experiment with this method, I recommend starting with your favorite cut of meat and marinade and going from there.

Canning

Your electric pressure cooker can be used for water-bath canning, but not for pressure canning. The USDA warns against using the electric pressure cooker for pressure canning because it can be challenging to produce enough pressure to kill off bacteria. You will want to can high-acid foods such as fruit, vegetables, pickles, and jams only.

When you are performing a water-bath can in your electric pressure cooker, follow these simple steps:

1. Place water at the bottom of the inner pot.

2. Place the trivet over the water.

3. Place your warm sealed jars on the trivet.

4. Close the electric pressure cooker and secure the lid.

5. Turn the steam release handle to "venting."

6. Wait for the float valve to pop up; you should see a steady stream of steam escaping from the pressure cooker.

7. Keep the lid on until all the steam has been released and the float valve has popped back down.

8. Open the pressure cooker and carefully remove the jars from the inner pot using tongs.

9. Keep the jars at room temperature until they have cooled.

TROUBLESHOOTING

When you are new to electric pressure-cooking, you might run into barriers when you start even if you have read your manual from cover to cover. Here is a list of common issues that might crop up and how to solve them:

Burn notices: If you see the "burn" notice show up on your control panel, various things could have happened.

» You may not have added enough cooking liquid. You need at least 1 cup of cooking liquid in the inner pot before pressure-cooking.

» If you are cooking a pasta dish, the water needs to cover the pasta entirely and you need to stir the pasta so that it doesn't cake on the bottom of the inner pot.

» If you used the sauté function before the pressure-cooking process, let the pot cool down for a few minutes before starting the cooking process. I always unplug my pot for at least 1 to 2 minutes.

» Always deglaze the inner pot after you sauté; the burn notice will turn on if there is any food stuck on the pot's bottom.

If you get a burn notice, cancel the pressure-cooking process. The fix might be as simple as adding more liquid or rotating the food to salvage the dish.

Sealing ring odor: Your sealing ring can retain an odor after cooking an aromatic soup, chili, or meat dish. Always wash your sealing ring after each use. You can also pick up an extra sealing ring and use one for savory dishes and one for desserts.

The electric pressure cooker is not sealing: Some of the reasons your pressure cooker may not be sealing include:

» The sealing ring is not installed correctly.

» The steam handle is in the venting position.

» There isn't enough steam to bring the pot to pressure. Make sure the recipe has enough liquid.

» The lid might not be properly closed.

» The float valve could be stuck because it needs to be cleaned out.

Steam from the quick release is damaging kitchen cabinets: Try to avoid letting out steam underneath your kitchen cabinets. The steam is hot and can damage the bottom of your kitchen cabinets.

You can:

» Set the pressure cooker on a kitchen island, if you have one.

» Try to let out steam near the kitchen sink, which generally doesn't have any cabinets above it.

» Keep the pressure cooker on a separate rack or shelf with no kitchen cabinets above it.

Float valve either won't fall or won't rise: Take it out and clean it.

Proteins are not cooked all the way through: When you cook a large piece of meat, it might not cook all the way through. Here are some tips to avoid this problem:

» If you're pressed for time, cut your protein into smaller pieces.

» When cooking a larger piece of meat than recommended in the recipe, add a few more minutes to the cooking time.

» Don't worry if it's not cooked all the way through! You can always put it back in and cook it for a few more minutes.

THE RECIPES IN THIS BOOK

This book includes many dishes that will help new electric pressure cooker users get the hang of this versatile kitchen tool. This book consists of some of the easiest and most popular recipes one can make in an electric pressure cooker. Each chapter has one essential dish—such as steel-cut oats, beans, risotto, and pulled pork—as well as two or more other recipes that are variations on these basic dishes. The essential dishes are a great place to start if you're new to electric pressure cooking.

Each recipe in this book has labels at the top to help you plan out your meals. In addition to identifying the **essential dishes,** you can also easily scan to see which recipes are **under 30 minutes, under an hour, worth the wait,** or **one-pot meals**. And for dietary concerns, appropriate recipes are also labeled as **dairy-free, gluten-free, vegan,** and **vegetarian**. At the end of the recipes, you will also find tips on ingredients, suggestions for variations to try, or recommendations for what to pair the recipe with to make a meal. And for anyone who wants to meal prep, check out the storage information.

At the top of each recipe, you will also find "at a glance" information about the prep time, cook time, release method, and total time. **Prep time** includes preliminary steps such as mixing, browning, whisking, and sautéing, as well as any steps that occur after pressure-cooking, such as reducing a sauce or folding a finishing ingredient (such as butter or cheese) into the cooked dish. **Cook time** refers specifically to the time under pressure—i.e., the number of minutes that you enter into the control panel. **Total time** is prep time + time under pressure + release time + the 5 to 10 minutes needed for the cooker to come up to pressure. I've tried to be as accurate as possible with all the information in these recipes, but the timing may vary depending on a number of factors, including differences among pressure cooker models.

Now that you know the fundamentals of how an electric pressure cooker works and the proper electric pressure cooker terminology, it's time to turn the page and start cooking.

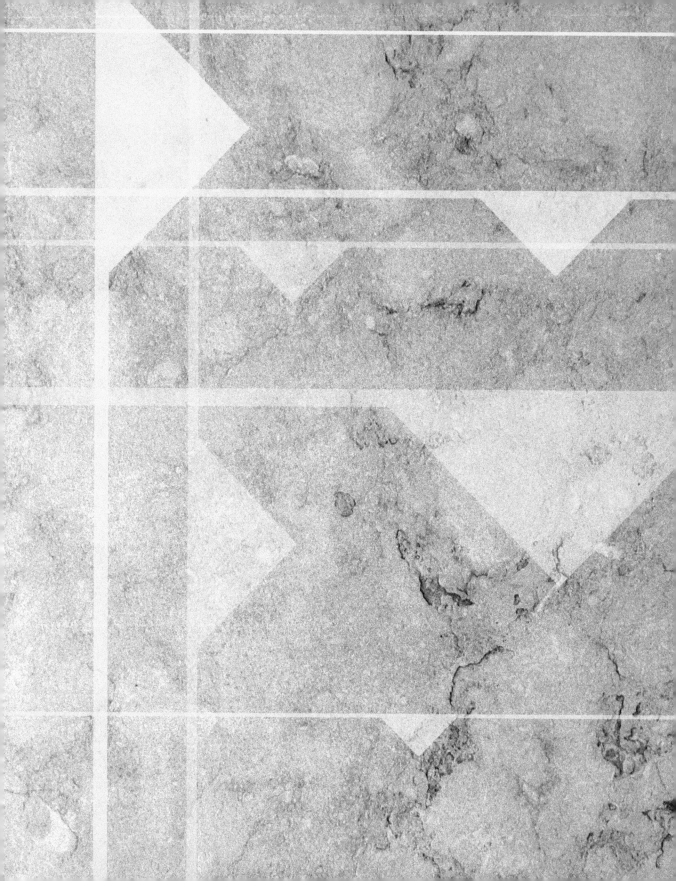

2 Breakfast

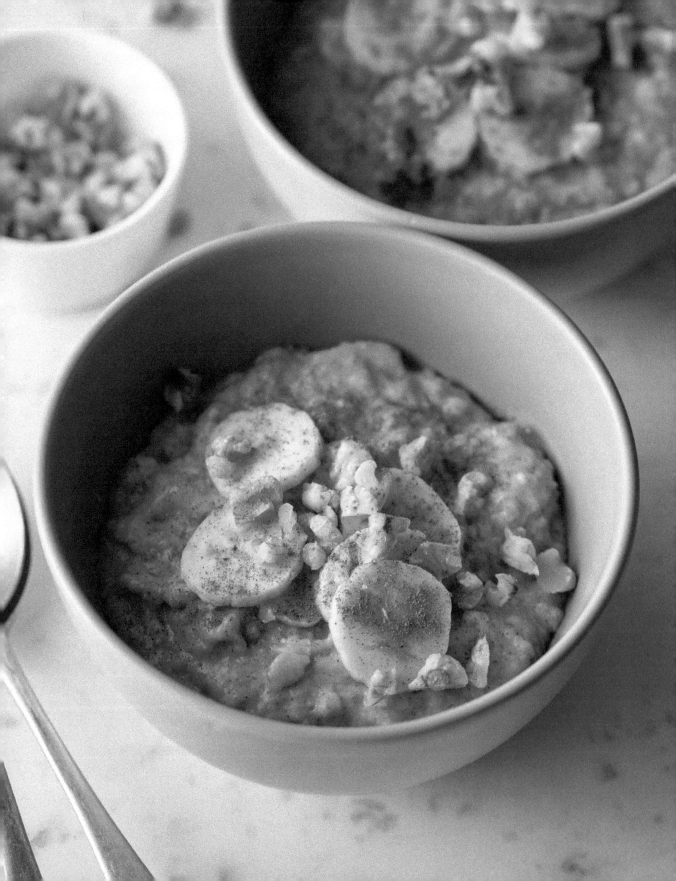

Creamy Banana-Nut Steel-Cut Oats

SERVES 4 TO 6
PREP TIME: 5 MINUTES • COOK TIME: 4 MINUTES • TOTAL TIME: 30 MINUTES
PRESSURE RELEASE: NATURAL
GLUTEN-FREE, ONE-POT MEAL, UNDER AN HOUR, VEGETARIAN

This recipe tastes exactly like banana bread but takes a fraction of the time. Steel-cut oats are a healthy breakfast option that will come together in minutes. This oatmeal is kid-pleasing and a nourishing way for families to start the day.

3½ cups whole milk

1 cup steel-cut oats

2 bananas, sliced

¼ cup packed light brown sugar

1 teaspoon sea salt

1 teaspoon pure vanilla extract

½ teaspoon ground cinnamon

½ cup chopped walnuts

1. In the inner pot, combine the milk, steel-cut oats, bananas, brown sugar, salt, vanilla, and cinnamon. Stir all the ingredients together.

2. Secure the lid and cook on high pressure for 4 minutes, then allow the pressure to naturally release for at least 10 minutes (as the oats will continue cooking during this time).

3. Remove the lid, stir the oats, and let stand for 5 minutes to thicken. Stir in the walnuts and serve.

INGREDIENT TIP: Avoid using overly ripe bananas in this recipe.

Creamy Blueberry-Lemon Steel-Cut Oats

SERVES 4 TO 6
PREP TIME: 5 MINUTES • COOK TIME: 4 MINUTES • TOTAL TIME: 30 MINUTES
PRESSURE RELEASE: NATURAL
ESSENTIAL RECIPE, GLUTEN-FREE, ONE-POT MEAL, UNDER AN HOUR,
VEGETARIAN

After your family tries these delectable steel-cut oats, you will never micro-wave store-bought oatmeal packets again. Steel-cut oats are a less processed version of rolled oats. They are chewy and nutty and reheat wonderfully. Pressure cooker steel-cut oats make a healthy, budget-friendly breakfast.

3½ cups whole milk

1 cup steel-cut oats

1 cup blueberries

¼ cup sugar

1 teaspoon sea salt

1 teaspoon grated lemon zest

1 teaspoon pure vanilla extract

Optional garnishes: blueberries, bananas, or nuts

1. In the inner pot, combine the milk, steel-cut oats, blueberries, sugar, salt, lemon zest, and vanilla.

2. Secure the lid and cook on high pressure for 4 minutes, then allow the pressure to naturally release for at least 10 minutes (as the oats will continue cooking during this time).

3. Remove the lid, stir the oats, and let stand for 5 minutes to thicken before serving. Garnish with blueberries, bananas, or nuts, if desired.

RECIPE TOOLBOX: If you want your oats creamier, add an additional ½ cup of milk.

Oatmeal Cookie Steel-Cut Oats

SERVES 4 TO 6
PREP TIME: 5 MINUTES • COOK TIME: 4 MINUTES • TOTAL TIME: 30 MINUTES
PRESSURE RELEASE: NATURAL
GLUTEN-FREE, ONE-POT MEAL, UNDER AN HOUR, VEGETARIAN

This dish is the perfect breakfast for the holidays. The oats turn out sweet, chewy, and nutty, just like an oatmeal cookie. You can make them quickly on a weekday morning, and they will keep your belly happy until lunch.

2 cups whole milk

1½ cups water

1 cup steel-cut oats

½ cup raisins

¼ cup packed light brown sugar

1 teaspoon sea salt

1 teaspoon pure vanilla extract

½ teaspoon ground cinnamon

½ cup chopped walnuts (optional)

1. In the inner pot, combine the milk, water, steel-cut oats, raisins, brown sugar, salt, vanilla, and cinnamon.

2. Secure the lid and cook on high pressure for 4 minutes, then allow the pressure to naturally release.

3. Remove the lid, stir the oats, and let stand for 5 minutes to thicken before serving. Garnish with walnuts, if desired.

INGREDIENT TIP: This recipe is best made with pure vanilla instead of imitation vanilla extract. I use Kirkland brand pure vanilla extract.

Soft-Boiled Eggs

MAKES 4 TO 6 EGGS
PREP TIME: 2 MINUTES • COOK TIME: 2 MINUTES • TOTAL TIME: 10 MINUTES
PRESSURE RELEASE: QUICK
DAIRY-FREE, GLUTEN-FREE, UNDER 30 MINUTES, VEGETARIAN

A properly cooked soft-boiled egg is the perfect addition to your breakfast toast, a delicious protein for your quick weekday salad, or the finishing touch to a burger, bowl of pasta, or sandwich. A soft-boiled egg also makes a great healthy snack any time of the day, so it is fabulous that you can make a soft-boiled egg in 10 minutes from start to finish.

1 cup water

4 to 6 large eggs

1. Pour the water into the inner pot and insert the trivet. Place the eggs on the trivet.

2. Secure the lid and cook on high pressure for 2 minutes, then quick release the pressure and remove the lid.

3. Remove the eggs from the pot and immediately run them under cold water.

4. Peel and serve.

> **MEAL PLANNING TIP:** Soft-boiled eggs can be a great protein to add to many recipes. Try them on top of Peanut Noodles (page 126).

Hard-Boiled Eggs

MAKES 6 TO 10 EGGS
PREP TIME: 2 MINUTES • COOK TIME: 5 MINUTES • TOTAL TIME: 20 MINUTES
PRESSURE RELEASE: NATURAL
DAIRY-FREE, GLUTEN-FREE, UNDER 30 MINUTES, VEGETARIAN

Hard-boiled eggs make great fillings for breakfast sandwiches. They're perfect on top of a Cobb salad, and of course, they can be whipped into egg salad for lunch. Best of all, hard-boiled eggs turn out perfectly when cooked in a pressure cooker, and the process couldn't be more straightforward.

1 cup water
6 to 10 large eggs

1. Pour the water into the inner pot and insert the trivet. Place the eggs on the trivet.

2. Secure the lid and cook on high pressure for 5 minutes. Allow the pressure to naturally release for 5 minutes, then quick release the remaining pressure and remove the lid.

3. Remove the eggs from the pot and immediately run under cold water.

4. Peel and serve.

STORAGE: Hard-boiled eggs can be refrigerated for up to 5 days.

MENU PLANNING TIP: You can add hard-boiled eggs as the protein to Coconut-Curry Rice with Cauliflower (page 127).

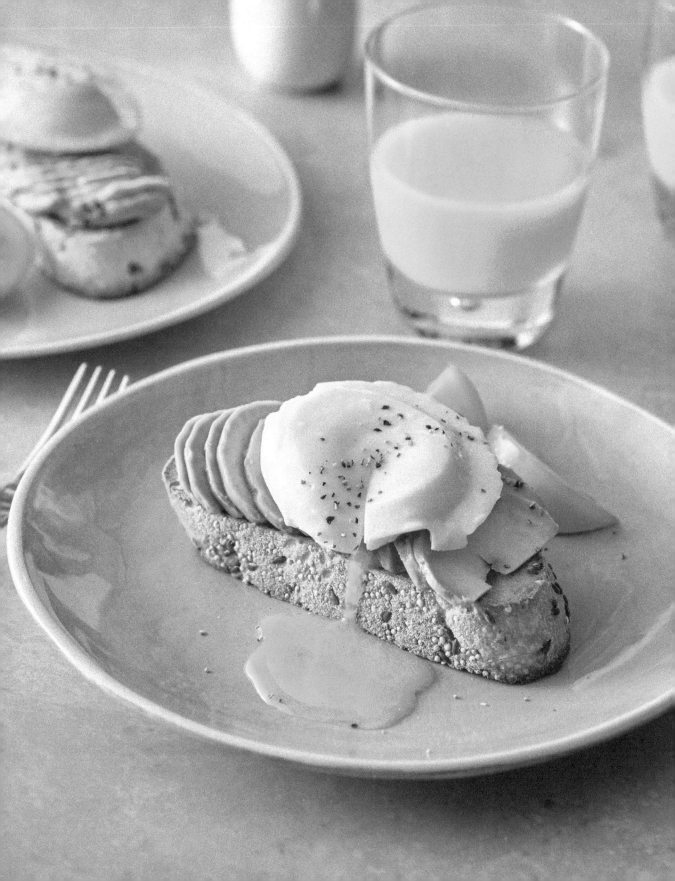

Perfect Poached Eggs

SERVES 4 TO 6
PREP TIME: 5 MINUTES • COOK TIME: 4 MINUTES • TOTAL TIME: 15 MINUTES
PRESSURE RELEASE: QUICK
DAIRY-FREE, GLUTEN-FREE, UNDER 30 MINUTES, VEGETARIAN

Once I discovered this hands-off and easy cooking method for multiple poached eggs in the electric pressure cooker, I never cooked them the traditional way again. Pressure cooker poached eggs are perfectly soft. I enjoy serving these on toast with slices of Canadian bacon or with flavorful topping combinations like Hummus (page 50) and sliced tomatoes or avocado, sea salt, and fresh lemon juice. This recipe uses silicone egg bite molds, but you can also use ramekins or small mason jars.

1 cup water

Nonstick cooking spray or olive oil

4 to 6 large eggs

1. Pour the water into the inner pot and insert the trivet.

2. Mist a silicone egg bite mold with cooking spray or grease with olive oil. Crack one egg into each section of the egg mold. Set the mold on the trivet.

3. Secure the lid and cook on high pressure for 2 to 3 minutes, then quick release the pressure and remove the lid.

4. Remove the trivet and mold. Use a spoon to gently scoop out each egg. Serve immediately.

MEAL PLANNING TIP: Poached eggs taste delicious as a protein over Vegan Black Bean Burrito Bowls (page 119).

Italian Poached Eggs

SERVES 4 TO 6
PREP TIME: 5 MINUTES • COOK TIME: 1 MINUTE • TOTAL TIME: 15 MINUTES
PRESSURE RELEASE: NATURAL
GLUTEN-FREE, ONE-POT MEAL, UNDER 30 MINUTES, VEGETARIAN

This simple dish of runny eggs poached in marinara sauce tastes delicious on a piece of crusty bread. With a one-minute cooking time, this meal will delight your family not only for breakfast but also for lunch or dinner.

1 cup water

2 cups store-bought marinara sauce

6 large eggs

2 tablespoons half-and-half

⅓ cup shredded Parmesan cheese

⅓ cup shredded mozzarella cheese

1. In the inner pot, combine the water and marinara sauce. One at a time, crack the eggs into a small bowl and gently add each egg, one at a time, onto the surface of the marinara sauce. Drizzle the half-and-half over the eggs.

2. Secure the lid and cook on high pressure for 1 minute. Allow the pressure to naturally release for 3 minutes, then quick release the remaining pressure and remove the lid.

3. Top the eggs with the cheeses and serve.

MENU PLANNING TIP: These Italian Poached Eggs also taste great on Parmesan Polenta (page 71).

Ricotta Egg Bites

MAKES 7 EGG BITES
PREP TIME: 5 MINUTES • COOK TIME: 8 MINUTES • TOTAL TIME: 35 MINUTES
PRESSURE RELEASE: NATURAL
GLUTEN-FREE, UNDER AN HOUR, VEGETARIAN

Egg bites are all the rage, and my kids love them. These tasty morsels became popular after they were introduced at a national coffee chain. The good news is you can make them at home and save money. These egg bites have a velvety texture and taste creamy and delicious. They store beautifully in the refrigerator for several days, although I doubt they will last that long. I like to use a silicone egg bite mold for this recipe, but they work in ramekins, mason jars, or silicone cupcake holders.

1 cup water

Oil or nonstick cooking spray

8 large eggs

1 cup ricotta cheese

1 teaspoon sea salt

1 teaspoon herbes de Provence

1. Pour the water into the inner pot and insert the trivet.

2. Lightly oil or mist a silicone egg bite mold (or ramekins or silicone cupcake holders).

3. In a medium bowl, whisk together the eggs, ricotta, salt, and herbes de Provence.

4. Pour the mixture into the wells of the egg bite mold, cover with either the lid or foil, and place the mold on the trivet.

5. Secure the lid and cook on high pressure for 8 minutes, then allow the pressure to naturally release. Press cancel.

6. Remove the lid and carefully remove the egg bites. Serve hot.

STORAGE: Refrigerate in a sealed container for up to 5 days or freeze for up to 2 months.

SWITCH IT UP: Add ham, sausage, peppers, or any favorite ingredients to create different flavors!

Ramekin Cinnamon Coffee Cakes

MAKES 5 CAKES
PREP TIME: 10 MINUTES • COOK TIME: 6 MINUTES • TOTAL TIME: 25 MINUTES
PRESSURE RELEASE: QUICK
UNDER 30 MINUTES, VEGETARIAN

These perfectly spiced treats come together in minutes and taste as heavenly as the cinnamon coffee cake from your favorite coffee shop.

For the batter

1 cup all-purpose flour

⅓ cup granulated sugar

1 teaspoon ground cinnamon

½ teaspoon sea salt

½ teaspoon baking powder

½ teaspoon baking soda

1 cup yogurt

4 tablespoons (½ stick) butter, melted

1 large egg

1 teaspoon pure vanilla extract

Vegetable oil or nonstick cooking spray

1 cup water

For the topping

2 tablespoons light brown sugar

2 tablespoons chopped walnuts

1 tablespoon butter

½ teaspoon ground cinnamon

To make the batter

1. In a large bowl, mix the flour, granulated sugar, cinnamon, salt, baking powder, and baking soda until well blended. Add the yogurt, melted butter, egg, and vanilla and stir to combine.

2. Lightly oil 5 (2-inch) ramekins (or coat with non-stick cooking spray) and divide the batter among the ramekins, filling each one almost to the top.

To make the topping

3. In a small bowl, stir together the brown sugar, chopped walnuts, butter, and cinnamon.

4. Place a spoonful of topping in each ramekin and cover them with aluminum foil.

5. Pour the water into the inner pot and insert the trivet. Arrange the ramekins on the trivet.

6. Secure the lid and cook on high pressure for 6 minutes, then quick release the pressure and remove the lid.

7. Use an oven mitt or tongs to remove the ramekins, uncover, and serve.

STORAGE: Refrigerate in a sealed container for up to 5 days.

MENU PLANNING TIP: These cakes are delicious for holiday brunch and pair well served alongside Hash Brown Crustless Quiche (page 44).

Hash Brown Crustless Quiche

SERVES 4 TO 6
PREP TIME: 5 MINUTES • COOK TIME: 20 MINUTES • TOTAL TIME: 40 MINUTES
PRESSURE RELEASE: NATURAL
GLUTEN-FREE, ONE-POT MEAL, UNDER AN HOUR

This quiche, cooked in a small springform pan, requires no prep ahead of time and comes together in just minutes. Egg dishes made in an electric pressure cooker cook evenly and are perfectly steamed every time. This sausage-and-cheese-packed quiche is a filling crowd-pleaser. You can easily adapt the ingredients to make this a family favorite.

4 breakfast sausage links, chopped into ½-inch pieces

1 cup water

8 large eggs

1½ cups frozen shredded hash brown potatoes (no need to thaw)

½ cup shredded Cheddar cheese

¼ cup whole milk

1 teaspoon seasoning salt

1. Select sauté and let the inner pot heat up for 2 minutes.

2. Add the sausage and sauté for about 5 minutes, or until it is cooked all the way through. Remove the sausage and set aside. Rinse the pot and scrub to remove any browned bits, then return the pot to the pressure cooker.

3. Pour the water into the inner pot and insert the trivet.

4. In a medium bowl, combine the eggs, frozen hash browns, cheese, cooked breakfast sausage, milk, and seasoning salt until well mixed.

5. Pour the egg mixture into a 7-inch springform pan and set the pan on the trivet.

6. Secure the lid and cook on high pressure for 15 minutes. Allow the pressure to naturally release for 10 minutes, then quick release any remaining pressure and remove the lid. Press cancel.

7. Remove the trivet and springform pan from the pot. Release the sides of the springform pan and serve.

STORAGE: Refrigerate in a sealed container for up to 5 days or freeze for 1 to 4 months.

SWITCH IT UP: You can replace the breakfast sausage with chorizo for a spicier egg casserole.

3 Beans, Vegetables, and Grains

Black Beans

SERVES 6 TO 8
PREP TIME: 5 MINUTES • COOK TIME: 30 MINUTES • TOTAL TIME: 1 HOUR
15 MINUTES
PRESSURE RELEASE: NATURAL
DAIRY-FREE, ESSENTIAL RECIPE, GLUTEN-FREE, VEGAN, WORTH THE WAIT

Black beans taste delicious in chili, burrito bowls, tacos, and salads. Once you realize how easy it is to cook black beans in your electric pressure cooker, you will never buy canned beans again. All you need to do is add all the ingredients to the inner pot and hit the "bean-chili" button. Home-cooked dried beans are lower in sodium and taste better than canned beans. Although no soaking is necessary, you can shorten the cooking time a bit if you do (see Ingredient Tip).

6 cups water
2 cups dried black beans
1 tablespoon onion powder
2 teaspoons sea salt

1. In the inner pot, combine the water, beans, onion powder, and salt.

2. Secure the lid and cook on high pressure for 30 minutes, then allow the pressure to naturally release for at least 30 minutes (as the beans will continue cooking during this time). Press cancel.

3. Remove the lid, drain the excess liquid from the beans, rinse, and serve.

STORAGE: Refrigerate in a sealed container for up to 5 days or freeze for up to 6 months.

INGREDIENT TIP: If you soak the beans before cooking them, reduce the cooking time by 10 minutes. This will work with any of the bean recipes in this book.

Lentils

SERVES 6 TO 8

PREP TIME: 2 MINUTES • COOK TIME: 8 MINUTES • TOTAL TIME: 45 MINUTES

PRESSURE RELEASE: NATURAL

DAIRY-FREE, GLUTEN-FREE, UNDER AN HOUR, VEGAN, WORTH THE WAIT

Lentils are a great staple to keep in your pantry. They're inexpensive, versatile, and protein-packed, making them a popular choice in many vegetarian dishes. They're also delicious in soups, curries, and casseroles. Cooking lentils in the electric pressure cooker is incredibly easy and they turn out delicious.

1¾ cups water

1 cup dried brown lentils

1 tablespoon olive oil

½ teaspoon sea salt

1 bay leaf

1 shallot, finely chopped

1. In the inner pot, combine the water, lentils, olive oil, salt, bay leaf, and shallot.

2. Secure the lid and cook on high pressure for 8 minutes, then allow the pressure to naturally release. Press cancel.

3. Remove the lid, discard the bay leaf, and serve.

STORAGE: Refrigerate in a sealed container for up to 5 days or freeze for up to 6 months.

SWITCH IT UP: Cook the lentils in broth instead of water for added flavor.

Hummus

SERVES 6 TO 8

PREP TIME: 5 MINUTES • COOK TIME: 30 MINUTES • TOTAL TIME: 1 HOUR

PRESSURE RELEASE: NATURAL

DAIRY-FREE, GLUTEN-FREE, VEGAN, WORTH THE WAIT

Making hummus in the pressure cooker is a game-changer. In my opinion, the best tasting hummus is smooth, lemony, and a little salty. Cooking dried chickpeas instead of using store-bought canned beans results in perfect-tasting hummus.

4 cups water

1 cup dried chickpeas

¼ cup olive oil

2 tablespoons tahini

1 tablespoon freshly squeezed lemon juice

1 teaspoon sea salt

1. In the inner pot, combine the water and dried chickpeas.

2. Secure the lid and cook on high pressure for 30 minutes, then allow the pressure to naturally release. Press cancel.

3. Remove the lid. Drain the chickpeas and transfer to a blender or food processor.

4. Add the olive oil, tahini, lemon juice, and salt and pulse until the hummus is smooth. Add a little more olive oil and blend further if you want it creamier.

5. Transfer to a serving dish and serve.

STORAGE: Refrigerate in a sealed container for up to 5 days.

COOK IT SLOW: Dried chickpeas can also be made in a slow cooker. Combine the dried chickpeas and water in a slow cooker and cook on low for 6 to 8 hours. Drain the chickpeas and make the hummus as directed above.

Pinto Beans

SERVES 6 TO 8
PREP TIME: 5 MINUTES • COOK TIME: 30 MINUTES • TOTAL TIME: 1 HOUR
15 MINUTES
PRESSURE RELEASE: NATURAL
DAIRY-FREE, GLUTEN FREE, VEGAN, WORTH THE WAIT

The combination of pinto beans and onions can't be beat. These Pinto Beans taste lovely as an accompaniment to any Southwestern-inspired dish such as tacos, burritos, burrito bowls, enchiladas, casseroles, and salads. I love adding all my favorite toppings to these beans to turn them into a stand-alone meal.

6 cups water

2 cups dried pinto beans

1 onion, chopped

2 teaspoons sea salt

2 teaspoons ground cumin

2 teaspoons smoked paprika

1 teaspoon chili powder

Optional toppings

Sour cream

Cilantro

Queso fresco cheese

Garden Salsa (page 231)

1. In the inner pot, combine the water, beans, onion, salt, cumin, smoked paprika, and chili powder.

2. Secure the lid and select the "bean/chili" mode, or cook on high pressure for 30 minutes. Allow the pressure to naturally release for at least 30 minutes (as the beans will continue cooking during this time). Press cancel.

3. Open the lid and drain the beans. Serve with your favorite toppings.

STORAGE: Refrigerate in a sealed container for up to 5 days or freeze for up to 6 months.

MENU PLANNING TIP: These Pinto Beans taste excellent alongside Tropical Salsa Chicken Breasts (page 144).

Cowboy Baked Beans

SERVES 6 TO 8

PREP TIME: 10 MINUTES • COOK TIME: 40 MINUTES • TOTAL TIME: 1 HOUR
5 MINUTES

PRESSURE RELEASE: NATURAL

DAIRY-FREE, GLUTEN-FREE, WORTH THE WAIT

These hearty baked beans are my go-to summer party side dish. They are flavor-packed and such a crowd-pleaser. Baked beans traditionally involve cooking dried navy beans for a long time, but with this recipe you can be liberated from your kitchen while your electric pressure cooker does all the work. Also, no soaking is necessary.

2 cups dried navy beans

5 cups water

1 cup brewed coffee

1 onion, chopped

3 bacon slices, chopped

½ cup barbecue sauce

¼ cup packed light brown sugar

2 tablespoons brown mustard

1 tablespoon Worcestershire sauce

1 teaspoon apple cider vinegar

1. In the inner pot, combine the beans, water, coffee, onion, bacon, barbecue sauce, brown sugar, mustard, Worcestershire sauce, and vinegar.

2. Secure the lid and select "bean/chili" mode, or cook on high pressure for 40 minutes. Allow the pressure to naturally release. Press cancel.

3. Remove the lid. If you have excess liquid, you may want to use the sauté setting to thicken the beans to your preference.

4. Serve hot.

STORAGE: Refrigerate in a sealed container for up to 5 days.

MENU PLANNING TIP: Cowboy Baked Beans taste great with Large-Batch Smoky Barbecue Pork Chop Sandwiches (page 172).

Italian White Beans with Lemon and Rosemary

SERVES 6 TO 8
PREP TIME: 5 MINUTES • COOK TIME: 30 MINUTES • TOTAL TIME: 1 HOUR
15 MINUTES
PRESSURE RELEASE: NATURAL
DAIRY-FREE, GLUTEN-FREE, VEGAN, WORTH THE WAIT

These lemon and rosemary–scented white beans are so versatile. They taste amazing on salads or on a piece of crusty bread and are fabulous as a side dish with any Italian entrée. This one-step cooking procedure in your electric pressure cooker creates a dish that your family will love.

3 cups water

2 cups dried great northern beans

3 shallots or 1 small onion, chopped

1 teaspoon sea salt

2 garlic cloves, minced

1 teaspoon dried rosemary

2 tablespoons olive oil

2 tablespoons freshly squeezed lemon juice

1. In the inner pot, combine the water, beans, shallots, salt, garlic, rosemary, olive oil, and lemon juice.

2. Secure the lid and select the "bean-chili" mode, or cook on high pressure for 30 minutes. Allow the pressure to naturally release. Press cancel.

3. Remove the lid and serve hot.

STORAGE: Refrigerate in a sealed container for up to 5 days.

Refried Beans

SERVES 6 TO 8
PREP TIME: 5 MINUTES • COOK TIME: 35 MINUTES • TOTAL TIME: 1 HOUR
15 MINUTES
▶ **PRESSURE RELEASE:** NATURAL
DAIRY-FREE, GLUTEN-FREE, VEGAN, WORTH THE WAIT

In my house, we always serve refried beans on taco night. After making these Refried Beans in your electric pressure cooker, you'll never go back to the can. This dish goes from dried to your table in just a little over an hour. They taste buttery and make delicious tacos, enchiladas, and burritos—and they're also wonderful straight out of the pot.

8 cups water

2 cups dried pinto beans

1 medium onion, chopped

1 garlic clove, minced

1 tablespoon freshly squeezed lime juice

1 tablespoon ground cumin

2 teaspoons sea salt

3 tablespoons vegetable oil

1. In the inner pot, combine the water, beans, onion, garlic, lime juice, cumin, and salt.

2. Secure the lid and select the "bean-chili" mode, or cook on high pressure for 30 minutes. Allow the pressure to naturally release. Press cancel.

3. Remove the lid, drain the beans, and return them to the pot. Add the oil, select sauté, and cook the beans for about 5 minutes while smashing them with a wooden spoon.

4. Serve hot.

STORAGE: Refrigerate in a sealed container for 3 to 4 days.

Sour Cream and Onion Mashed Potatoes

SERVES 6 TO 8
PREP TIME: 10 MINUTES • COOK TIME: 8 MINUTES • TOTAL TIME: 30 MINUTES
PRESSURE RELEASE: QUICK
GLUTEN-FREE, UNDER AN HOUR, VEGETARIAN

These mashed potatoes are rich, creamy, and filled with tangy onion flavor. They cook up fast and easy, making them a great weeknight side dish or stress-free accompaniment to a holiday meal. Cooking mashed potatoes in your electric pressure cooker means they are tender enough to be mashed easily without an electric mixer.

3 pounds Yukon Gold potatoes, peeled and halved

4 cups water

1 cup sour cream

4 tablespoons (½ stick) butter

¼ cup chopped scallions

1 tablespoon onion powder

Sea salt

Freshly ground black pepper

1. Place the potatoes in the inner pot and add the water, or enough to cover the potatoes by ¼ inch or so. If the potatoes are sticking up above the water, try rearranging them first to get them below the water level rather than adding more water.

2. Secure the lid and cook on high pressure for 8 minutes, then quick release the pressure and remove the lid. Press cancel.

3. Drain the potatoes in a colander and return them to the pot.

4. Stir in the sour cream, butter, scallions, onion powder, and salt and pepper to taste. Serve hot.

STORAGE: Refrigerate in a sealed container for up to 5 days.

MENU PLANNING TIP: These mashed potatoes taste great with Herbes de Provence Pork Chops (page 174).

Goat Cheese Creamed Spinach

SERVES 4
PREP TIME: 10 MINUTES • COOK TIME: 3 MINUTES • TOTAL TIME: 25 MINUTES
PRESSURE RELEASE: QUICK
GLUTEN-FREE, UNDER 30 MINUTES, VEGETARIAN

Creamed spinach is a tasty way to get a hefty serving of a healthy vegetable. This dish packs a lot of flavor, and it couldn't be easier to make. You simply steam the spinach in the pressure cooker's steamer basket for 0 minutes. When you choose a cooking time of 0 minutes, a soon as the pressure cooker achieves pressure, the pressure-cooking process will stop. Adding goat cheese to creamed spinach kicks it up a notch. I enjoy eating creamed spinach on a baked potato, accompanied by a pork chop or alongside eggs.

1 cup water
10 ounces baby spinach
1 shallot, chopped
2 ounces soft goat cheese
1 tablespoon olive oil
1 teaspoon minced garlic
1 teaspoon cornstarch
½ teaspoon ground nutmeg
1 tablespoon whole milk

1. Pour the water into the inner pot and insert a steamer basket. Place the spinach and chopped shallot into the steamer.

2. Secure the lid and cook on high pressure for 0 minutes (the cooker will come to pressure and immediately stop the pressure-cooking process), then quick release the pressure and remove the lid. Press cancel.

3. Drain the spinach and shallots in a colander. Return the spinach to the pressure cooker pot.

4. Select sauté. If your electric pressure cooker lets you choose a heat level for sauté, press low. Let the pot heat up (it can take up to 5 minutes if set on low). Add the goat cheese, olive oil, garlic, cornstarch, and nutmeg to the spinach. Sauté for about 3 minutes, or until the cornstarch thickens

the spinach and the goat cheese is creamed throughout the spinach.

5. Stir in the milk to combine. Serve hot.

STORAGE: Refrigerate in a sealed container for up to 3 days.

MENU PLANNING TIP: This creamed spinach tastes wonderful with Perfect Poached Eggs (page 39) on top.

Cauliflower-Potato Mash

SERVES 4

PREP TIME: 10 MINUTES • COOK TIME: 5 MINUTES • TOTAL TIME: 25 MINUTES

PRESSURE RELEASE: QUICK

GLUTEN-FREE, UNDER 30 MINUTES, VEGETARIAN

Adding tender cauliflower to classic mashed potatoes creates a side dish that pleases the whole family. Parents love it because it's full of healthy cauliflower and kids love it because it's creamy, comforting, and delicious. A win for everyone!

1 cup water

1½ pounds Yukon Gold potatoes (4 medium), peeled and halved

1 medium head cauliflower, quartered

¼ cup whole milk

2 ounces cream cheese

1 tablespoon butter

1 tablespoon fresh or dried chopped chives

2 garlic cloves, minced

Sea salt

Freshly ground black pepper

1. Pour the water into the inner pot and insert the trivet or a steamer basket. Arrange the potatoes and cauliflower on the trivet or in the basket.

2. Secure the lid and cook on high pressure for 5 minutes, then quick release the pressure and remove the lid. Press cancel.

3. Drain the potatoes and cauliflower and return them to the pot. Add the milk, cream cheese, butter, chives, and garlic. Season to taste with salt and pepper, mix to your desired consistency, and serve.

STORAGE: Refrigerate in a sealed container for up to 5 days.

MENU PLANNING TIP: This mash tastes excellent as a side dish for Large-Batch Smoky Barbecue Pork Chop Sandwiches (page 172).

Buttered Rum Baby Carrots

SERVES 4 TO 6
PREP TIME: 10 MINUTES • COOK TIME: 8 MINUTES • TOTAL TIME: 25 MINUTES
PRESSURE RELEASE: QUICK
GLUTEN-FREE, UNDER 30 MINUTES, VEGETARIAN

These lovely carrots are quite a treat and are an easy side dish to bring to any holiday gathering. They are sweet and rich-tasting, and you can whip them up in just a few minutes. This is a two-step recipe: First, you quickly cook the carrots in the pressure cooker, then you use the sauté function to make the quick and easy buttered rum sauce.

1 cup water

1 (16-ounce) bag baby carrots

1 teaspoon sea salt

4 tablespoons (½ stick) butter

¼ cup half-and-half or whole milk

1 shot or 3 tablespoons spiced rum

2 tablespoons light brown sugar

1 teaspoon pure vanilla extract

1. Pour the water into the inner pot and insert a steamer basket. Add the baby carrots and sea salt to the steamer.

2. Secure the lid and cook on high pressure for 3 minutes, then quick release the pressure and remove the lid. Press cancel.

3. Drain the carrots in a colander.

4. Return the pot to the pressure cooker and select sauté. Add the butter, half-and-half, spiced rum, brown sugar, and vanilla. Stir for about 5 minutes to thicken the sauce.

5. Add the carrots, stir to coat, and serve.

STORAGE: Refrigerate in a sealed container for up to 5 days.

MENU PLANNING TIP: These baby carrots make a great side dish for Turkey Breast with Shallot Gravy (page 155).

Salted Baby Potatoes

SERVES 4 TO 6
PREP TIME: 5 MINUTES • COOK TIME: 16 MINUTES • TOTAL TIME: 35 MINUTES
PRESSURE RELEASE: NATURAL
GLUTEN-FREE, UNDER AN HOUR, VEGETARIAN

Any occasion, any time of year is the perfect time to make these wonderful potatoes. This side dish uses few ingredients and makes an excellent accompaniment to beef, pork, chicken, or fish. The potatoes cook up velvety on the inside and crispy on the outside.

1 cup water

1 (1½-pound) bag baby potatoes, washed and pierced with a fork

1 tablespoon butter

1 tablespoon olive oil

1 tablespoon coarse sea salt

1 teaspoon dried thyme

1. Pour the water into the inner pot and insert the trivet or steamer basket. Place the potatoes on the trivet or in the basket. Place the butter on top of the potatoes.

2. Secure the lid and cook on high pressure for 12 minutes. Allow the pressure to naturally release for 10 minutes, then quick release the remaining pressure and remove the lid. Press cancel.

3. Remove the potatoes and trivet or steamer. Pour out the water and return the potatoes to the pot.

4. Add the olive oil, salt, and thyme to the pot, select sauté, and sauté the potatoes for 4 minutes, or until they are coated with salt and crispy. Serve hot.

STORAGE: Refrigerate in a sealed container for up to 1 week.

MENU PLANNING TIP: These potatoes pair well with Smoky Barbecue Ribs (page 177).

Cheesy Broccoli

SERVES 4 TO 6
PREP TIME: 5 MINUTES • COOK TIME: 1 MINUTE • TOTAL TIME: 15 MINUTES
PRESSURE RELEASE: QUICK
GLUTEN-FREE, UNDER 30 MINUTES, VEGETARIAN

Cheesy Broccoli is an easy weeknight side dish that my kids love. Learning how to cook this vegetable in my electric pressure cooker was a game-changer because this method produces perfectly al dente broccoli. This recipe is salty, buttery, and cheesy, and I promise that your family will regularly ask for it.

1 cup water

3 cups broccoli florets

½ cup shredded Cheddar cheese

1 tablespoon butter

1 teaspoon sea salt

1. Pour the water into the inner pot and insert a steamer basket. Add the broccoli to the basket.

2. Secure the lid and cook on high pressure for 1 minute, then quick release the pressure and remove the lid. Press cancel.

3. Transfer the broccoli to a medium serving bowl. Add the cheese, butter, and sea salt and toss to coat. Serve hot.

STORAGE: Refrigerate in a sealed container for up to 3 days.

INGREDIENT TIP: I recommend shredding your own cheese instead of buying packaged shredded cheese. Packaged cheese can contain a coating that prevents it from melting as smoothly.

Steamed Sugar Snap Peas with Herbs

SERVES 4
PREP TIME: 5 MINUTES • COOK TIME: 2 MINUTES • TOTAL TIME: 10 MINUTES
PRESSURE RELEASE: QUICK
DAIRY-FREE, GLUTEN-FREE, UNDER 30 MINUTES, VEGAN

Sugar snap peas are a favorite vegetable in my home. We grow them in our garden every summer and buy them year-round for various dishes. They are sweet, and when I add a few of my favorite herbs, it balances the flavors in this side dish. Sugar snap peas can be steamed in the electric pressure cooker in mere minutes, and they turn out tender but still slightly crunchy.

⅓ cup water

8 ounces sugar snap peas

1 teaspoon olive oil

1 shallot, chopped

1 teaspoon chopped
fresh dill

1 teaspoon chopped
fresh tarragon

1 teaspoon freshly squeezed
lemon juice

Pinch sea salt

1. Pour the water into the inner pot and insert a steamer basket or trivet. Place the sugar snap peas in the basket or on the trivet.

2. Secure the lid and cook on low pressure for 0 minutes, then quick release the pressure and remove the lid. Press cancel.

3. Drain the snap peas into a colander.

4. Return the pot to the pressure cooker and add the olive oil, shallot, dill, tarragon, lemon juice, and salt. Select sauté. Add the sugar snap peas and cook for about 2 minutes, or until the shallots are softened. Serve hot.

MENU PLANNING TIP: These peas are wonderful with the Three-Cheese Risotto (page 102) and the Creamy French Mustard Chicken (page 143).

Sweet Potato Mash with Marshmallow Creme

SERVES 4 TO 6

PREP TIME: 5 MINUTES • COOK TIME: 8 MINUTES • TOTAL TIME: 25 MINUTES

PRESSURE RELEASE: QUICK

GLUTEN-FREE, UNDER 30 MINUTES, VEGETARIAN

Sweet potatoes are a kid-pleasing side dish and a great choice to bring to any special gathering. My family enjoys this sweet potato mash throughout the year. The sweet potatoes become so tender when cooked in an electric pressure cooker that no mixer will be necessary to mash these up. Adding the marshmallow takes this dish over the top.

1 cup water

2 pounds sweet potatoes (about 6 medium), peeled and halved

2 tablespoons butter

1 teaspoon sea salt

1 teaspoon pure vanilla extract

½ cup marshmallow creme

1. Pour the water into the inner pot and insert a steamer basket or trivet. Place the sweet potatoes into the steamer or on the trivet.

2. Secure the lid and cook on high pressure for 8 minutes, then quick release the pressure and remove the lid. Press cancel.

3. Drain the sweet potatoes into a colander and return them to the pot.

4. Add the butter, salt, and vanilla and mash with a fork. Gently stir the marshmallow creme into the warm sweet potatoes right before serving.

STORAGE: Refrigerate in a sealed container for up to 3 days.

MENU PLANNING TIP: These sweet potatoes taste excellent alongside Turkey Breast with Shallot Gravy (page 155).

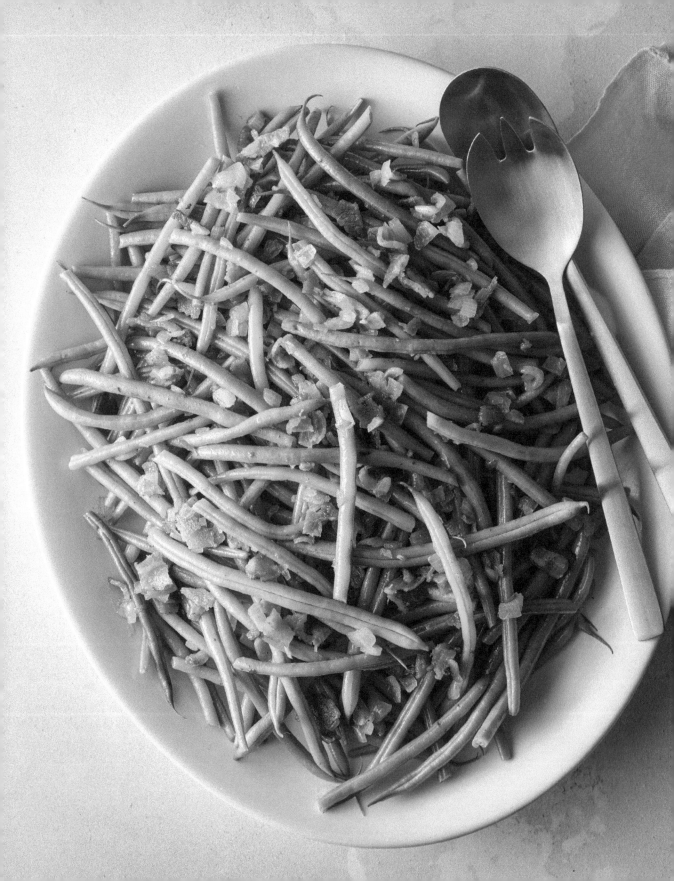

Green Beans with Shallots and Bacon

SERVES 4 TO 6

PREP TIME: 10 MINUTES • COOK TIME: 7 MINUTES • TOTAL TIME: 20 MINUTES

PRESSURE RELEASE: QUICK

DAIRY-FREE, GLUTEN-FREE, UNDER 30 MINUTES

If you regularly buy fresh green beans like I do, then this is the recipe for you. The beans steam in just a few short minutes and taste wonderful when paired with smoky bacon and sweet shallots. It is a side dish fancy enough to serve for a holiday meal, but quick enough for a busy weeknight.

1 cup water

1 pound green beans, trimmed

2 bacon slices, chopped

2 shallots, chopped

½ teaspoon sea salt

1. Pour the water into the inner pot and insert a steamer basket or trivet. Place the green beans in the steamer or on the trivet.

2. Secure the lid and cook on high pressure for 2 minutes, then quick release the pressure and remove the lid. Press cancel.

3. Remove the steamer or trivet and pour the water out of the pot.

4. Return the pot to the pressure cooker and select sauté. Add the bacon, shallots, and salt. (It might take up to 2 minutes for the pot to heat up.) Sauté for about 5 minutes, or until the bacon crisps up and the shallots are browned.

5. Add the bacon-shallot mixture (including the bacon fat) to the green beans. Serve hot.

STORAGE: Refrigerate in a sealed container for up to 5 days.

SWITCH IT UP: For sweeter green beans, add 1 tablespoon of brown sugar with the shallots and bacon.

Simple Corn on the Cob

SERVES 4 TO 6
PREP TIME: 2 MINUTES • COOK TIME: 2 MINUTES • TOTAL TIME: 15 MINUTES
PRESSURE RELEASE: QUICK
GLUTEN-FREE, UNDER 30 MINUTES, VEGETARIAN

There is nothing quite like an ear of corn, perfectly cooked and dripping with butter. Corn on the cob is perfect when made in an electric pressure cooker. This is my go-to summer side dish because the corn is sweet, easy, healthy, local, and my kids are obsessed with it.

1 cup water

4 ears corn, husked and halved

2 tablespoons butter

1 teaspoon salt

1. Pour the water into the inner pot and insert the trivet. Place the corn on the trivet.

2. Secure the lid and cook on high pressure for 2 minutes, then quick release the pressure and remove the lid. Press cancel.

3. Remove the corn. Spread with butter and sprinkle the salt on each ear of corn while still warm.

MENU PLANNING TIP: Corn on the cob is an excellent side dish to go with Sloppy Joes (page 182).

Farro

SERVES 4 TO 6
PREP TIME: 5 MINUTES • COOK TIME: 14 MINUTES • TOTAL TIME: 35 MINUTES
PRESSURE RELEASE: NATURAL
DAIRY-FREE, UNDER AN HOUR, VEGAN

There are many fabulous reasons to become acquainted with farro, a type of wheat from Northern Italy, and learn how to cook it in your electric pressure cooker. Farro is nutty, chewy, and full of protein and fiber. Use this versatile supergrain as a base for grain bowls or as an accompaniment to Mediterranean dishes.

1 tablespoon olive oil
2 cups farro, rinsed
3½ cups water
1 garlic clove
1 bay leaf
1 teaspoon sea salt

1. Pour the olive oil into the inner pot, then add the farro. Select sauté and toast the farro for 2 minutes.

2. Press cancel to turn off the heating element and add the water, garlic, bay leaf, and sea salt to the pot.

3. Secure the lid and cook on high pressure for 12 minutes. Allow the pressure to naturally release for 10 minutes, then quick release the remaining pressure. Press cancel.

4. Remove the lid. If the farro looks watery, don't worry, it will thicken in a few minutes. Discard the bay leaf, let the farro rest for 5 minutes, then serve.

STORAGE: Refrigerate in a sealed container for up to 5 days or freeze for up to 6 months.

RECIPE TOOLBOX: Toasting the farro before starting the pressure-cooking process enhances the flavor. I use this same technique in all of the risotto recipes in chapter 5.

Sticky Rice

SERVES 4 TO 6
PREP TIME: 2 MINUTES • COOK TIME: 12 MINUTES • TOTAL TIME: 35 MINUTES
PRESSURE RELEASE: NATURAL
DAIRY-FREE, GLUTEN-FREE, UNDER AN HOUR, VEGAN

Electric pressure cookers produce perfect tender sticky rice—every time. If you only used your electric pressure cooker to cook rice, your investment would still be worth it. The cooking time under pressure for this rice is only 12 minutes, and it tastes delightful with stir-fries, curries, and as a stand-alone side dish.

1 tablespoon sesame oil

3 cups water

2 cups jasmine rice

1 teaspoon sea salt

1. Coat the bottom of the inner pot with the sesame oil, then add the water, rice, and salt.

2. Secure the lid and select the "rice" mode, or cook on high pressure for 12 minutes. Allow the pressure to naturally release for at least 10 minutes (as the rice continues cooking during that time).

3. Remove the lid and serve.

STORAGE: Refrigerate in a sealed container for up to 5 days or freeze for up to 6 months.

INGREDIENT TIP: This recipe works for jasmine rice and long-grain Thai rice. To cook brown rice, see Brown Rice (page 72).

Mango-Ginger Sticky Rice

SERVES 4 TO 6
PREP TIME: 2 MINUTES • COOK TIME: 12 MINUTES • TOTAL TIME: 35 MINUTES
PRESSURE RELEASE: NATURAL
DAIRY-FREE, GLUTEN-FREE, UNDER AN HOUR, VEGAN

Adding mango and ginger is a delicious way to switch up your rice game.
I used canned mango with the juice as a liquid element in this recipe for an
extra hit of sweetness. You can eat this rice alongside stir-fries, in sushi bowls,
and as a delicious side dish. This recipe works with jasmine rice and long-grain
Thai rice.

1 tablespoon sesame oil

2 cups water

2 cups jasmine rice

2 cups canned mango with
the mango juice

2 teaspoons ground ginger

1. Coat the bottom of the inner pot with the sesame
   oil (move the oil around with a spatula), then
   add the water, rice, mango, mango juice, and
   ground ginger.

2. Secure the lid and select the "rice" mode, or cook
   on high pressure for 12 minutes. Allow the pressure to naturally release. Press cancel.

3. Remove the lid and serve.

STORAGE: Refrigerate in a sealed container for
up to 5 days or freeze for up to 6 months.

RECIPE TOOLBOX: If you are in a rush, you can use
the quick-release method. The longer you let the
rice naturally release, the stickier it will be.

Wild Rice with Apples and Shallots

SERVES 4 TO 6
PREP TIME: 5 MINUTES • COOK TIME: 32 MINUTES • TOTAL TIME: 55 MINUTES
PRESSURE RELEASE: NATURAL
DAIRY-FREE, GLUTEN-FREE, UNDER AN HOUR, VEGAN

Wild rice is the perfect side dish to serve when it's cold outside. I like to serve it alongside turkey, and it also tastes great in soups and casseroles. Cooking wild rice can be intimidating, but not when you own an electric pressure cooker. This flavorful recipe is a great side dish for any winter holiday gathering.

1 tablespoon olive oil

3 shallots or 1 small onion, chopped

½ cup shredded peeled Granny Smith apples

3 cups water

2 cups wild rice

1 teaspoon sea salt

1 teaspoon dried thyme

1. Select sauté and let the pot heat up for 2 minutes.

2. Add the olive oil, shallots, and apples and sauté for 2 to 3 minutes, until the shallots are translucent.

3. Add the water, wild rice, sea salt, and thyme.

4. Secure the lid and cook on high pressure for 30 minutes, then allow the pressure to naturally release. Press cancel.

5. Remove the lid and serve.

STORAGE: Refrigerate in a sealed container for up to 5 days or freeze for up to 6 months.

SWITCH IT UP: This wild rice is a great gluten-free stuffing option for holiday meals. When I make it as a stuffing, I add ½ pound of pork sausage to it, cooking the sausage at the same time as the apples and shallots.

Parmesan Polenta

SERVES 4
PREP TIME: 3 MINUTES • COOK TIME: 5 MINUTES • TOTAL TIME: 30 MINUTES
PRESSURE RELEASE: NATURAL
GLUTEN-FREE, UNDER AN HOUR, VEGETARIAN

Polenta is a creamy and buttery Northern Italian dish that costs mere pennies a serving but is found in the finest Italian restaurants because it tastes that good. Making polenta using the stovetop method requires attentiveness and a lot of whisking, which is why I love the hands-off approach of cooking it in my electric pressure cooker instead.

4 cups water

1 cup cornmeal

1 tablespoon butter

1 teaspoon minced garlic

1 teaspoon sea salt

½ cup grated
Parmesan cheese

1. In the inner pot, whisk together the water, cornmeal, butter, garlic, and salt.

2. Secure the lid and cook on high pressure for 5 minutes, then allow the pressure to naturally release. Press cancel.

3. Remove the lid and stir in the Parmesan and serve.

INGREDIENT TIP: This recipe works best with fine cornmeal, such as the Quaker brand. Coarse cornmeal will work but is going to be a tad lumpy.

Brown Rice

SERVES 6

PREP TIME: 3 MINUTES • COOK TIME: 25 MINUTES • TOTAL TIME: 50 MINUTES

PRESSURE RELEASE: NATURAL

DAIRY-FREE, GLUTEN-FREE, UNDER AN HOUR, VEGAN

Cooked brown rice is a great ingredient to keep around for dinner leftovers, a filling and delicious lunch, soups, stir-fries, and heaped in tacos. Brown rice turns out nutty and fluffy when cooked in an electric pressure cooker. This cooking method is much less labor-intensive than cooking brown rice on the stovetop.

1 tablespoon olive oil

2 cups short or long-grain brown rice

2 cups water

2 teaspoons sea salt

1. Pour the olive oil into the inner pot and add the rice, water, and sea salt.

2. Secure the lid and cook on high pressure for 25 minutes, then allow the pressure to naturally release. Press cancel.

3. Remove the lid and serve.

STORAGE: Refrigerate in a sealed container for up to 5 days or freeze for up to 6 months.

INGREDIENT TIP: This recipe is for short-grain or long-grain brown rice. Avoid using quick-cook rice.

Middle Eastern Couscous

SERVES 4 TO 6
PREP TIME: 5 MINUTES • COOK TIME: 5 MINUTES • TOTAL TIME: 20 MINUTES
PRESSURE RELEASE: QUICK
UNDER 30 MINUTES, VEGETARIAN

Couscous is super easy to prepare in the electric pressure cooker. This version pairs deliciously with roasted vegetables and tastes terrific on any Mediterranean salad. Couscous with za'atar seasoning is a great way to switch up the flavors at home and is an excellent potluck dish.

2½ cups water

2 cups Israeli
(pearl) couscous

2 tablespoons butter or
olive oil

1 shallot or
⅓ onion, chopped

1 teaspoon freshly squeezed
lemon juice

1 teaspoon za'atar seasoning

1. Pour the water into the inner pot. Add the couscous, butter, shallot, lemon juice, and za'atar seasoning.

2. Secure the lid and cook on high pressure for 5 minutes, then quick release the pressure and remove the lid. Press cancel.

3. Stir together to evenly distribute the seasonings and serve.

STORAGE: Refrigerate in a sealed container for up to 5 days.

SWITCH IT UP: Electric pressure cooker couscous is great with a variety of different seasonings. Greek seasonings, Italian seasonings, and herbes de Provence would all taste delicious in place of the za'atar in this couscous.

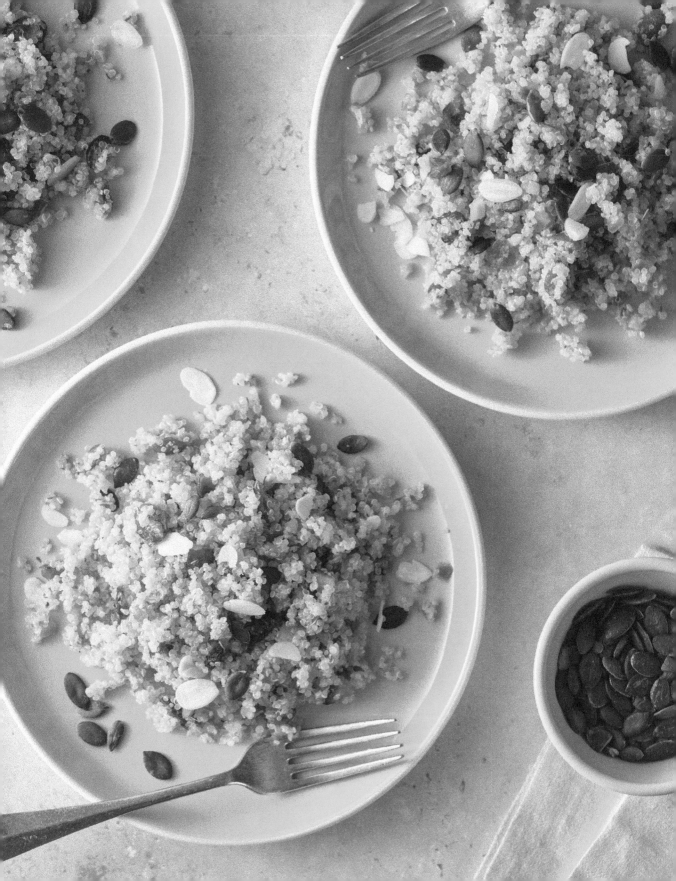

Easy Quinoa with Cranberries and Herbs

SERVES 4 TO 6
PREP TIME: 2 MINUTES • COOK TIME: 1 MINUTE • TOTAL TIME: 15 MINUTES
PRESSURE RELEASE: NATURAL
DAIRY-FREE, GLUTEN-FREE, UNDER 30 MINUTES, VEGAN

Quinoa turns out perfectly fluffy when cooked in an electric cooker; it will not disappoint. This dish is studded with sweet cranberries, and the savory herbs taste divine. It is perfect for cold weather or as a cozy side dish to any holiday spread.

2 cups quinoa

2 cups vegetable broth, store-bought or homemade (page 222)

½ cup dried cranberries

½ cup chopped red onion

1 teaspoon sea salt

1 teaspoon dried sage

1 teaspoon dried thyme

¼ cup pumpkin seeds (optional)

¼ cup slivered almonds (optional)

1. In the inner pot, combine the quinoa, vegetable broth, dried cranberries, onion, sea salt, sage, and thyme.

2. Secure the lid and cook on high pressure for 1 minute, then allow the pressure to naturally release. Press cancel.

3. Remove the lid and serve, garnished with pumpkin seeds and almonds, if desired.

STORAGE: Refrigerate in a sealed container for up to 5 days or freeze for up to 6 months.

INGREDIENT TIP: This recipe works with white, black, red, or tri-color quinoa.

4 Soups and Stews

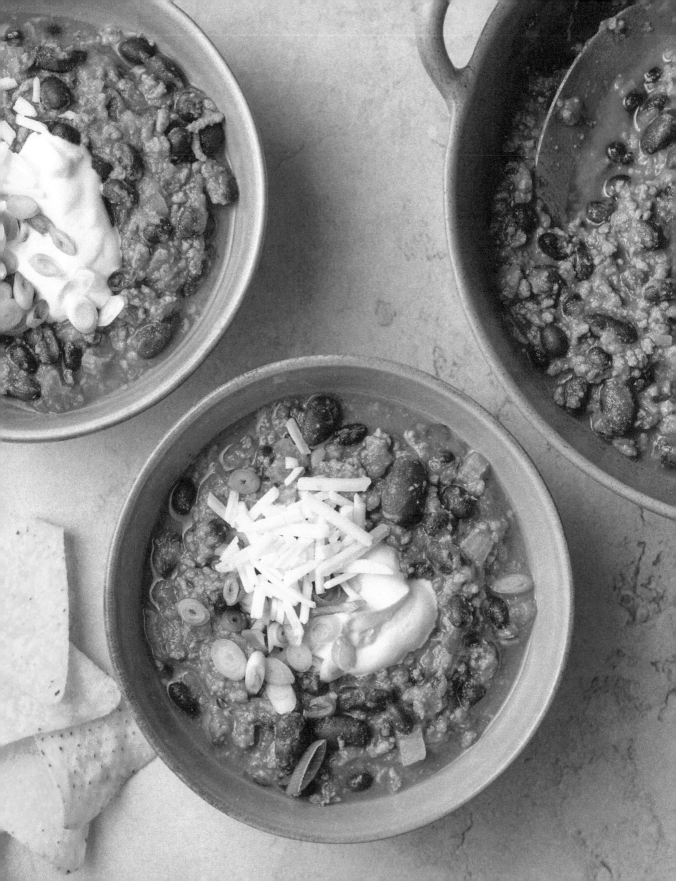

Basic Beef Chili

SERVES 6
PREP TIME: 8 MINUTES • COOK TIME: 22 MINUTES • TOTAL TIME: 45 MINUTES
PRESSURE RELEASE: NATURAL
DAIRY-FREE, ESSENTIAL RECIPE, GLUTEN-FREE, ONE-POT MEAL,
UNDER AN HOUR

There is nothing as comforting as a warm bowl of chili with toppings galore. Chili is one of my favorite meals to make in my electric pressure cooker. This recipe tastes like it simmered in a slow cooker all day long, but it's easy enough to throw together in just 45 minutes.

1 tablespoon olive oil

1 small onion, chopped

¼ cup chopped celery

1 pound ground beef

1 (28-ounce) can crushed tomatoes

1 tablespoon tomato paste

1 cup water

1 (15-ounce) can black beans, drained and rinsed

1 (15-ounce) can kidney beans, drained and rinsed

1 tablespoon chili powder

1 tablespoon ground cumin

1 teaspoon dried oregano

1 teaspoon garlic powder

1 teaspoon cayenne pepper (optional)

1. Select sauté and let the pot heat up for 2 minutes.

2. Add the olive oil, onion, and celery and sauté for 2 minutes, or until translucent.

3. Add the ground beef and brown for 3 minutes. You do not need to cook it all the way through.

4. Add the tomatoes, tomato paste, water, black beans, kidney beans, chili powder, cumin, oregano, garlic powder, and cayenne (if using), stirring to combine.

5. Secure the lid and cook on high pressure for 12 minutes, then allow the pressure to naturally release. Press cancel and remove the lid.

6. Select sauté and cook for about 5 minutes to thicken the chili slightly. Serve hot.

STORAGE: Refrigerate in a sealed container for up to 5 days or freeze for up to 6 months.

RECIPE TOOLBOX: I often make a big batch of chili so I can have leftovers to make Cheesy Chili Mac (page 180).

Minestrone Chili

SERVES 6

PREP TIME: 8 MINUTES • COOK TIME: 20 MINUTES • TOTAL TIME: 45 MINUTES
PRESSURE RELEASE: NATURAL
DAIRY-FREE, GLUTEN-FREE, ONE-POT MEAL, UNDER AN HOUR

This mouthwatering, Italian-style dish is a combination of two of my favorite meals—minestrone soup and beef chili. The addition of all the vegetables makes this a healthy weeknight dinner with many comforting flavors. Your family will surely give this chili two thumbs up.

1 tablespoon olive oil

1 small onion, chopped

¼ cup chopped celery

2 garlic cloves, minced

1 pound ground beef

1 (20-ounce) can crushed tomatoes

1 (15-ounce) can great northern beans, drained and rinsed

2 cups chopped zucchini

2 cups baby spinach

1 cup frozen cut green beans (no need to thaw)

1 cup chopped carrots

1 cup water

1 teaspoon dried rosemary

2 bay leaves

Parmesan rind (optional)

1. Select sauté and let the pot heat up for 2 minutes.

2. Pour the olive oil into the inner pot, then add the onion, celery, and garlic. Sauté for 2 minutes, or until translucent.

3. Add the ground beef and brown for 3 minutes. You do not need to cook it all the way through.

4. Add the tomatoes, beans, zucchini, spinach, green beans, carrots, water, rosemary, bay leaves, and Parmesan rind (if using).

5. Secure the lid and cook on high pressure for 12 minutes, then let the pressure naturally release. Press cancel and remove the lid.

6. Select sauté and cook for 2 to 3 minutes to thicken the chili.

7. Discard the bay leaves and rind (if using) and serve.

STORAGE: Refrigerate in a sealed container for up to 5 days or freeze for up to 6 months.

SWITCH IT UP: To make this vegetarian, replace the beef with 2 more 15-ounce cans of beans.

Baked Beans Chili

SERVES 6
PREP TIME: 8 MINUTES • COOK TIME: 20 MINUTES • TOTAL TIME: 45 MINUTES
PRESSURE RELEASE: NATURAL
DAIRY-FREE, GLUTEN-FREE, ONE-POT MEAL, UNDER AN HOUR

This chili is a great recipe to make if you have leftover baked beans around, and my kids love it. The sweet baked beans combine beautifully with the chili seasonings.

1 tablespoon vegetable oil

1 small onion, chopped

½ cup chopped celery

1 teaspoon minced garlic

1 pound ground beef

1 (28-ounce) can baked beans or 3 cups Cowboy Baked Beans (page 52)

1 (20-ounce) can crushed tomatoes

1 (15-ounce) can black beans, drained and rinsed

1 cup tomato juice

1 tablespoon chili powder

1 tablespoon ground cumin

1 teaspoon dried oregano

1. Select sauté and add the olive oil to the inner pot. Let the pot and the oil heat up for about 2 minutes.

2. Add the onion, celery, and garlic and cook for about 2 minutes, or until the onion is translucent.

3. Add the ground beef and brown for 3 minutes. You do not need to cook it all the way through.

4. Add the baked beans, tomatoes, black beans, tomato juice, chili powder, cumin, and oregano to the pot.

5. Secure the lid and cook on high pressure for 12 minutes, then let the pressure naturally release. Press cancel and remove the lid.

6. Select sauté and cook for an additional 2 to 3 minutes to thicken the chili. Serve hot.

STORAGE: Refrigerate in a sealed container for up to 5 days or freeze for up to 6 months.

COOK IT SLOW: This recipe can be easily adapted for a slow cooker. Brown the ground beef on the stovetop and add it to a slow cooker along with the other ingredients. Cook on low for 6 hours.

Chicken Salsa Soup with Lime

SERVES 6
PREP TIME: 5 MINUTES • COOK TIME: 10 MINUTES • TOTAL TIME: 35 MINUTES
PRESSURE RELEASE: NATURAL
DAIRY-FREE, GLUTEN-FREE, ONE-POT MEAL, UNDER AN HOUR

Chicken Salsa Soup with Lime is an easy one-step recipe that cooks up fast and is made with ingredients that are probably already in your pantry or freezer. Lime juice adds brightness and creates a succulent and flavorful dish. Though I prefer fresh lime juice, I always keep a bottle in my fridge in case I don't have any limes handy. This recipe is an easy, quick dinner or a great soup to eat throughout the week for lunch.

1 pound boneless, skinless chicken breasts

6 cups chicken stock, store-bought or homemade (page 223)

1½ cups Garden Salsa (page 231)

1 small onion, chopped

4 garlic cloves, minced

½ cup frozen corn kernels

¼ cup freshly squeezed lime juice

1. In the inner pot, combine the chicken, chicken stock, salsa, onion, garlic, corn, and lime juice.

2. Secure the lid and cook on high pressure for 10 minutes, then let the pressure naturally release. Press cancel.

3. Remove the lid. Transfer the chicken to a bowl and shred using two forks. Return the chicken to the soup and serve.

STORAGE: Refrigerate in a sealed container for up to 5 days or freeze for up to 6 months.

INGREDIENT TIP: Frozen chicken can easily be used in this recipe. No thawing is necessary.

Southwestern Lentil Soup

SERVES 6
PREP TIME: 10 MINUTES • COOK TIME: 8 MINUTES • TOTAL TIME: 30 MINUTES
PRESSURE RELEASE: QUICK
DAIRY-FREE, GLUTEN-FREE, ONE-POT MEAL, UNDER AN HOUR, VEGAN

This filling soup is a great meatless alternative to traditional Southwestern chicken and beef soups. You will enjoy a great, healthy, budget-friendly dish that warms you up on cold nights and makes a great lunch. This soup is a "dump and press start" recipe and is vegan but will please meat eaters and non–meat eaters alike!

4 cups vegetable broth, store-bought or homemade (page 222), or water

1 cup dried lentils or 2 cups cooked lentils

1 (20-ounce) can crushed tomatoes

1 cup frozen corn kernels

1 small onion, chopped

2 garlic cloves, minced

1 tablespoon chili powder

1 tablespoon ground cumin

1 teaspoon dried oregano

1. In the inner pot, combine the broth, lentils, tomatoes, corn, onion, garlic, chili powder, cumin, and oregano.

2. Secure the lid and cook on high pressure for 8 minutes, then quick release the pressure and remove the lid. Press cancel.

3. Serve hot.

STORAGE: Refrigerate in a sealed container for up to 5 days or freeze for up to 6 months.

INGREDIENT TIP: Both red and brown lentils will work great in this soup.

Black Bean Vegetable Soup

SERVES 6
PREP TIME: 10 MINUTES • COOK TIME: 8 MINUTES • TOTAL TIME: 30 MINUTES
PRESSURE RELEASE: QUICK
DAIRY-FREE, GLUTEN-FREE, ONE-POT MEAL, UNDER AN HOUR, VEGAN

The black beans and vegetables in this soup get a significant flavor boost from all the aromatics and the added lime juice. This meatless soup is high in protein, high in fiber, filled with vegetables, and seasoned perfectly, all while having a short ingredient list. The combination of creamy black beans, carrots, lime juice, and spices is delectable.

3 cups vegetable broth, store-bought or homemade (page 222), or water

2 cups cooked black beans, canned or homemade (page 48)

1 small onion, chopped

3 medium carrots, chopped

1 cup frozen corn kernels

1 (14.5-ounce) can fire-roasted diced tomatoes

2 garlic cloves, minced

2 tablespoons freshly squeezed lime juice

2 teaspoons ground cumin

1 teaspoon cayenne pepper

1 bay leaf

1. In the inner pot, combine the broth, black beans, onion, carrots, corn, tomatoes, garlic, lime juice, cumin, cayenne, and bay leaf.

2. Secure the lid and cook on high pressure for 8 minutes, then quick release the pressure and remove the lid. Press cancel.

3. Discard the bay leaf and serve.

STORAGE: Refrigerate in a sealed container for up to 5 days or freeze for up to 6 months.

SWITCH IT UP: If you like extra spice, add more cayenne or 1 chopped jalapeño pepper.

Lemon-Rosemary Chicken Noodle Soup

SERVES 6
PREP TIME: 5 MINUTES • COOK TIME: 12 MINUTES • TOTAL TIME: 30 MINUTES
PRESSURE RELEASE: QUICK
DAIRY-FREE, ONE-POT MEAL, UNDER AN HOUR

There is nothing quite like a piping hot bowl of chicken noodle soup on a winter day. Once you start adding lemon juice and rosemary to this dish, you won't go back. This soup tastes like the flavors have been blending for hours, but the cooking time is only 12 minutes. You will love the delicious aroma when you open up the pressure cooker.

2 cups chicken stock, store-bought or homemade (page 223)

2 cups water

2 cups egg noodles

1 pound boneless, skinless chicken breasts

⅓ cup freshly squeezed lemon juice

1 small onion, finely chopped

2 carrots, chopped

½ cup chopped celery

1 tablespoon olive oil

1½ teaspoons dried rosemary

1 teaspoon dried thyme

1. In the inner pot, combine the stock, water, egg noodles, chicken, lemon juice, onion, carrots, celery, oil, rosemary, and thyme.

2. Secure the lid and cook on high pressure for 12 minutes, then quick release the pressure and remove the lid. Press cancel.

3. Remove the chicken to a bowl and shred it using two forks. Return it to the soup and serve hot.

STORAGE: Refrigerate in a sealed container for up to 5 days or freeze for up to 6 months.

INGREDIENT TIP: If you prefer your noodles to be al dente, cook them separately right before serving. Divide them among bowls and ladle the soup over them.

Chicken Minestrone

SERVES 6
PREP TIME: 10 MINUTES • COOK TIME: 14 MINUTES • TOTAL TIME: 30 MINUTES
PRESSURE RELEASE: QUICK
DAIRY-FREE, GLUTEN-FREE, ONE-POT MEAL, UNDER AN HOUR

Packed full of vegetables and irresistible Italian flavors, Chicken Minestrone is the perfect healthy meal to serve at any time of the year. I love topping this quick-cooking soup with Parmesan cheese.

2 tablespoons olive oil

1 small onion,
finely chopped

3 garlic cloves, minced

4 medium Yukon Gold
potatoes, quartered

1 (28-ounce) can
crushed tomatoes

2 cups chicken stock,
store-bought or homemade
(page 223)

1 pound boneless, skinless
chicken thighs

1 cup frozen cut green beans
(no need to thaw)

1 medium zucchini, chopped

½ cup chopped celery

½ cup chopped carrots

1 tablespoon tomato paste

1 tablespoon
Italian seasoning

1. Select sauté and let the pot heat up for 2 minutes.

2. Add the olive oil, onion, and garlic and sauté for 2 minutes, or until the onion is translucent,

3. Add the potatoes, tomatoes, stock, chicken thighs, green beans, zucchini, celery, carrots, tomato paste, and Italian seasoning.

4. Secure the lid and cook on high pressure for 12 minutes, then quick release the pressure and remove the lid. Press cancel.

5. Remove the chicken to a bowl and shred it using two forks. Return the chicken to the soup and serve.

STORAGE: Refrigerate in a sealed container for up to 5 days or freeze for up to 6 months.

COOK IT SLOW: You can easily adapt this recipe for your slow cooker. Just add all the ingredients together to a slow cooker and cook on low for 4 to 6 hours. Shred the chicken as directed and return it to the soup.

Leftover Turkey and Leek Soup

SERVES 6

PREP TIME: 10 MINUTES • COOK TIME: 15 MINUTES • TOTAL TIME: 30 MINUTES

PRESSURE RELEASE: QUICK

GLUTEN-FREE, ONE-POT MEAL, UNDER AN HOUR

I have been hosting Thanksgiving for both sides of our family since I was 23 years old, which means that I am always on the lookout for new ways to use holiday leftovers. After a long day of cooking a holiday meal, it's nice to know you can create a round-two recipe with your leftover turkey that takes barely any time. Turkey and leeks taste especially great when cooked together in this hearty soup.

2 tablespoons butter

2 leeks, white part only, finely chopped

½ cup chopped celery

4 cups chicken stock, store-bought or homemade (page 223)

2 cups shredded cooked turkey

3 carrots, chopped

½ cup raw white rice

1 teaspoon herbes de Provence

1 bay leaf

1 cup heavy (whipping) cream

1. Select sauté and let the pot heat up for 2 minutes.

2. Add the butter, leeks, and celery and sauté for 2 to 3 minutes to soften.

3. Add the chicken stock, turkey, carrots, rice, herbes de Provence, and bay leaf.

4. Secure the lid and cook on high pressure for 12 minutes, then quick release the pressure and remove the lid. Press cancel.

5. Discard the bay leaf. Stir in the heavy cream and serve.

STORAGE: Refrigerate in a sealed container for up to 5 days.

INGREDIENT TIP: If you don't have heavy cream, you can use half-and-half or whole milk.

Ham Bone and Bean Soup

SERVES 6
PREP TIME: 15 MINUTES • COOK TIME: 14 MINUTES • TOTAL TIME: 45 MINUTES
PRESSURE RELEASE: NATURAL
GLUTEN-FREE, ONE-POT MEAL, UNDER AN HOUR

Ham Bone and Bean Soup is an excellent round-two recipe to make from leftovers. If you don't have a leftover ham bone, you can buy them from most butcher shops. My kids enjoy the rich flavor of ham broth, which tastes excellent with great northern beans' creaminess. I love our family tradition of making this soup every year after the holidays.

1 tablespoon butter

1 small onion, chopped

½ cup chopped celery

2 garlic cloves, minced

6 cups water

1 leftover ham bone

2 cups chopped
leftover ham

1 cup canned great northern
beans, drained and rinsed

3 carrots, chopped

1 cup frozen corn kernels
(no need to thaw)

1 cup frozen cut green beans
(no need to thaw)

1 teaspoon dried thyme

1 bay leaf

1. Select sauté and let the pot heat up for 2 minutes.

2. Add the butter, onion, and celery and sauté for 2 minutes, or until the onion is translucent.

3. Add the water, ham bone, ham, beans, carrots, corn, green beans, thyme, and bay leaf.

4. Secure the lid and cook on high pressure for 12 minutes, then allow the pressure to naturally release. Press cancel.

5. Remove the lid. Discard the ham bone and bay leaf. Serve hot.

STORAGE: Refrigerate in a sealed container for up to 5 days or freeze for up to 6 months.

SWITCH IT UP: This soup is fine without a ham bone. Just replace the water with chicken stock or vegetable broth.

Beef, Mushroom, and Barley Soup

SERVES 6

PREP TIME: 15 MINUTES • COOK TIME: 12 MINUTES • TOTAL TIME: 55 MINUTES

PRESSURE RELEASE: NATURAL

ONE-POT MEAL, UNDER AN HOUR

Over the years, this beef and grain–packed soup has become a family favorite because it is easy to whip up and mostly made with pantry and freezer staples. It is a budget-friendly dinner and also a great dish to serve at potlucks and parties.

3 cups beef stock, store-bought or homemade (page 224)

1 pound stewing beef, cut into 1-inch chunks

1 (28-ounce) can crushed tomatoes

1 (12-ounce) bag frozen mixed vegetables (no need to thaw)

1 cup pearl barley, rinsed

8 ounces baby bella mushrooms, washed and left whole

3 carrots, chopped

1 small onion, chopped

½ cup chopped celery

2 tablespoons Worcestershire sauce

1 tablespoon butter

1 garlic clove, minced

1 bay leaf

1. In the inner pot, combine the beef stock, beef, tomatoes, mixed vegetables, barley, mushrooms, carrots, onion, celery, Worcestershire sauce, butter, garlic, and bay leaf.

2. Secure the lid and cook on high pressure for 12 minutes, then allow the pressure to naturally release. Press cancel.

3. Remove the lid. Discard the bay leaf and serve.

STORAGE: Refrigerate in a sealed container for up to 5 days or freeze for up to 6 months.

SWITCH IT UP: For a vegetarian soup, replace the beef with another package of mushrooms and the beef stock with vegetable broth.

Chimichurri Beef Stew

SERVES 4 TO 6
PREP TIME: 15 MINUTES • COOK TIME: 16 MINUTES • TOTAL TIME: 55 MINUTES
PRESSURE RELEASE: NATURAL
GLUTEN-FREE, ONE-POT MEAL, UNDER AN HOUR

Adding zesty chimichurri to beef stew elevates the flavor of this classic comfort food. Chimichurri is an Argentinian condiment that I love for its depth of flavor. This recipe highlights the electric pressure cooker's knack for making inexpensive meat cuts tender and fantastic.

For the chimichurri

1 cup olive oil

1 cup flat-leaf parsley

¼ cup roughly chopped fresh oregano

¼ cup red wine vinegar

2 teaspoons minced garlic

Dash sea salt

Dash freshly ground black pepper

For the beef stew

1 tablespoon butter

1 small onion, chopped

½ cup chopped celery

1 pound stewing beef, large chunks halved

1 pound Yukon Gold potatoes, peeled and cut into ½-inch cubes

2 cups beef stock, store-bought or homemade (page 224)

4 carrots, chopped

To make the chimichurri

1. In a food processor, combine the olive oil, parsley, oregano, vinegar, garlic, salt, and pepper and pulse about five times. You want the sauce mixed, but not fully blended. Makes about 1½ cups.

To make the beef stew

2. Select sauté. Add the butter, onion, and celery and sauté for 2 minutes, or until the onion is translucent.

3. Add the beef and ¾ cup of the chimichurri and slightly sear the beef in the sauce for 2 minutes. Add the potatoes, beef stock, and carrots.

4. Secure the lid and cook on high pressure for 12 minutes, then allow the pressure to naturally release for at least 10 minutes (as the stew will continue cooking during that time). Press cancel.

5. Remove the lid. Serve garnished with a dollop of chimichurri on top. Any extra chimichurri will keep in the refrigerator for up to 2 weeks.

STORAGE: Refrigerate in a sealed container for up to 5 days or freeze for up to 6 months.

COOK IT SLOW: This recipe can be easily adapted for your slow cooker. Just sauté the onions ahead of time and add them to the slow cooker with the rest of the ingredients. Cook on low for 4 to 6 hours.

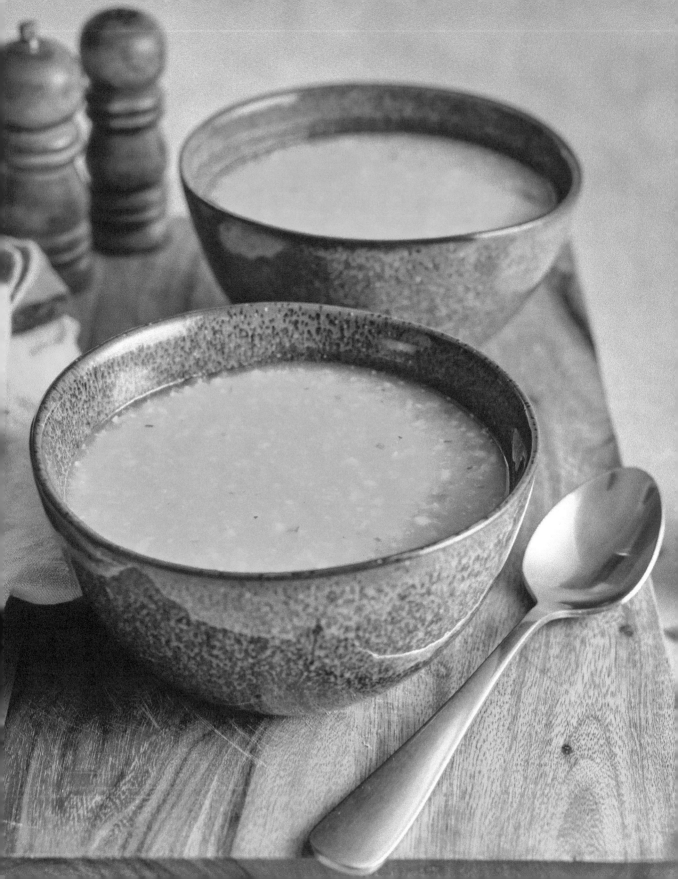

Butternut Squash and Corn Chowder with Bacon

SERVES 4 TO 6

PREP TIME: 10 MINUTES • COOK TIME: 10 MINUTES • TOTAL TIME: 30 MINUTES

PRESSURE RELEASE: QUICK

GLUTEN-FREE, ONE-POT MEAL, UNDER AN HOUR

Adding butternut squash to summery corn chowder results in an outrageously good soup that's a big hit with my family. The smoky bacon is the perfect foil for the sweetness of the corn and butternut squash. I pulse this soup with an immersion blender to make it creamy, but I leave a little texture. It is the perfect soup to enjoy during sweet corn season.

1 tablespoon butter

2 bacon slices, chopped

1 small onion, chopped

4 cups vegetable broth, store-bought or homemade (page 222)

2 (12-ounce) bags frozen corn kernels (no need to thaw)

1 medium butternut squash, peeled and cut into ½-inch cubes

½ teaspoon dried thyme

1 teaspoon dried chives

1. Select sauté. Add the butter, bacon, and onion to the pot and sauté for 2 minutes, or until the bacon is cooked and the onions are translucent.

2. Add the vegetable broth, corn, butternut squash, thyme, and chives to the pot.

3. Secure the lid and cook on high pressure for 8 minutes, then quick release the pressure and remove the lid. Press cancel.

4. Use an immersion blender to blend the soup, leaving a bit of texture (or transfer it to a stand blender in batches). Serve.

STORAGE: Refrigerate in a sealed container for up to 5 days or freeze for up to 6 months.

SWITCH IT UP: To make this soup vegan, replace the butter with olive oil and omit the bacon.

Garden Tomato Soup with Carrots

SERVES 6 TO 8
PREP TIME: 10 MINUTES • COOK TIME: 10 MINUTES • TOTAL TIME: 30 MINUTES
PRESSURE RELEASE: QUICK
DAIRY-FREE, GLUTEN-FREE, ONE-POT MEAL, UNDER AN HOUR, VEGAN

There is nothing quite like dunking a grilled cheese sandwich in a bowl of tomato soup. My family looks forward to a big batch of homemade tomato soup every summer when it's time to harvest tomatoes from our garden. High-quality canned tomatoes will also work well for this recipe. My secret ingredient for tomato soup has always been carrots, which naturally sweeten the dish and balance the acid in the tomatoes.

2 tablespoons olive oil

1 medium onion, chopped

2 garlic cloves, minced

10 to 12 medium tomatoes, chopped or 1 (28-ounce) can whole tomatoes

8 medium carrots, chopped

2 cups vegetable broth, store-bought or homemade (page 222)

6 fresh basil leaves

1 to 2 cups whole milk or heavy (whipping) cream (optional)

1. Select sauté and let the pot heat up for 2 minutes.

2. Pour the olive oil into the pot, then add the onions and garlic and sauté for 2 minutes, or until the onions are translucent.

3. Add the tomatoes, carrots, broth, and basil leaves.

4. Secure the lid and cook on high pressure for 8 minutes, then quick release the pressure and remove the lid. Press cancel.

5. Use an immersion blender to blend the soup (or transfer the soup to a stand blender in batches). If desired, stir in the milk before serving warm.

STORAGE: Refrigerate in a sealed container for up to 5 days or freeze for up to 6 months.

INGREDIENT TIP: If fresh tomatoes are not available, use good-quality canned peeled whole tomatoes: I recommend Hunt's, Cento, and Red Gold. All these brands should be easily found at your local grocery store.

Butternut Apple Cider Bisque

SERVES 4 TO 6
PREP TIME: 10 MINUTES • COOK TIME: 10 MINUTES • TOTAL TIME: 30 MINUTES
PRESSURE RELEASE: NATURAL
GLUTEN-FREE, ONE-POT MEAL, UNDER AN HOUR

Butternut squash soup is a staple at my mom's yearly Christmas Eve spread. This bisque is perfectly creamy, just sweet enough, and has only a tiny bit of spice. It will please adults and kids at your next holiday gathering or around the table on a weeknight.

1 tablespoon butter

1 small onion, chopped

1 tablespoon dried thyme

1 tablespoon dried sage

1 medium butternut squash, peeled and cut into ½-inch cubes (about 4 cups)

2 cups chicken stock, store-bought or homemade (page 223)

1 cup apple cider

1 cup whole milk or heavy (whipping) cream

1. Select sauté. Add the butter, onion, thyme, and sage and sauté for 2 minutes, or until the onions are translucent.

2. Add the butternut squash, chicken stock, and apple cider to the inner pot.

3. Secure the lid and cook on high pressure for 8 minutes, then allow the pressure to naturally release.

4. Open the vent at the top, remove the lid, and press cancel.

5. Use an immersion blender to blend the soup or transfer it to a blender in batches. Add the milk or cream right before serving.

STORAGE: Refrigerate in a sealed container for up to 5 days or freeze for up to 6 months.

INGREDIENT TIP: If apple cider is not available, you can use unsweetened apple juice. Add ½ teaspoon of cinnamon to help give the apple juice a little depth of flavor.

Cream of Shallot Soup

SERVES 6
PREP TIME: 10 MINUTES • COOK TIME: 15 MINUTES • TOTAL TIME: 30 MINUTES
PRESSURE RELEASE: QUICK
GLUTEN-FREE, ONE-POT MEAL, UNDER AN HOUR

This luscious shallot-packed soup is a cozy, simple meal to serve on a cold day. The ingredient list is short, but the flavor is huge. I like serving it with a side salad and a piece of crusty bread. It's also a great soup to whip up to replace the canned condensed soups in casseroles and noodles dishes.

3 tablespoons butter

10 shallots, chopped

1 teaspoon dried thyme

1 teaspoon dried rosemary

4 cups chicken stock, store-bought or homemade (page 223)

1 tablespoon cornstarch

½ cup heavy (whipping) cream or whole milk

1. Select sauté. Add the butter, shallots, thyme, and rosemary to the pot and sauté for 2 minutes, or until the onions are translucent.

2. Add the chicken stock.

3. Secure the lid and cook on high pressure for 8 minutes, then quick release the pressure and remove the lid. Press cancel.

4. Select sauté. Whisk in the cornstarch and cook for about 5 minutes to thicken the soup. Press cancel.

5. Use an immersion blender to blend the soup (or transfer it to a stand blender in batches). Stir in the cream and serve.

STORAGE: Refrigerate in a sealed container for up to 5 days.

COOK IT SLOW: Add all of the ingredients except the cream and cornstarch to a slow cooker and cook on low for 6 hours. Thirty minutes before it's done, use an immersion blender to blend the soup, then stir in the cream and cornstarch; it will thicken as it cooks for the last half hour.

Creamy Asparagus Soup with Bacon

SERVES 6

PREP TIME: 5 MINUTES • COOK TIME: 14 MINUTES • TOTAL TIME: 35 MINUTES

PRESSURE RELEASE: QUICK

GLUTEN-FREE, ONE-POT MEAL, UNDER AN HOUR

I enjoy making this soup during the springtime, when asparagus starts popping up. It is the perfect simple soup because it requires only a handful of ingredients but tastes amazing.

1 tablespoon butter

3 shallots or 1 small onion, chopped

2 bacon slices, chopped

1½ pounds thick asparagus spears, woody ends trimmed, halved

3 cups chicken stock, store-bought or homemade (page 223)

1 cup whole milk or heavy (whipping) cream

1. Select sauté. Add the butter, shallots, and bacon and sauté for 2 minutes, or until the shallots are translucent.

2. Add the asparagus and chicken stock.

3. Secure the lid and cook on high pressure for 12 minutes, then quick release the pressure and remove the lid. Press cancel.

4. Use an immersion blender to blend the soup (or transfer it to a stand blender in batches).

5. Stir in the milk right before serving.

STORAGE: Refrigerate in a sealed container for up to 5 days or freeze for up to 6 months.

SWITCH IT UP: To make this soup vegetarian, use vegetable broth instead of chicken stock and omit the bacon.

Creamy Carrot Soup

SERVES 6

PREP TIME: 5 MINUTES • COOK TIME: 10 MINUTES • TOTAL TIME: 25 MINUTES

PRESSURE RELEASE: QUICK

GLUTEN-FREE, ONE-POT MEAL, UNDER 30 MINUTES

Even the pickiest of eaters will enjoy this decadent soup. Carrots are incredibly sweet, and your kids will forget that they are eating a whole lot of vegetables. This soup calls for minimal ingredients, all of which you probably keep around, and will come together in no time.

2 tablespoons butter

1 large onion, chopped

2 pounds carrots, cut into ½-inch chunks

5 cups chicken stock, store-bought or homemade (page 223)

3 tablespoons freshly squeezed lemon juice

1 teaspoon dried thyme

1 cup heavy (whipping) cream or whole milk

1. Select sauté. Add the butter and onion and cook for 2 minutes, or until the onion is translucent.

2. Add the carrots, chicken stock, lemon juice, and thyme.

3. Secure the lid and cook on high pressure for 8 minutes, then quick release the pressure and remove the lid. Press cancel.

4. Use an immersion blender to blend the soup (or transfer it to a stand blender in batches).

5. Stir in the cream right before serving.

STORAGE: Refrigerate in a sealed container for up to 5 days or freeze for up to 6 months.

COOK IT SLOW: This recipe can easily be adapted to a slow cooker. Sauté the onions in the butter separately, then add them to the slow cooker along with the carrots, stock, lemon juice, and thyme. Cook on low for 4 to 6 hours. Add the cream right before serving.

Scandinavian Salmon Chowder

SERVES 6

PREP TIME: 15 MINUTES • COOK TIME: 20 MINUTES • TOTAL TIME: 45 MINUTES

PRESSURE RELEASE: NATURAL

GLUTEN-FREE, ONE-POT MEAL, UNDER AN HOUR

During the holiday season, my dad will serve us a few of the Scandinavian dishes that he grew up with. That tradition inspired this simple chowder. The rich salmon, buttery leeks, velvety potatoes, and tangy dill make for a knockout flavor combination. When you lift the electric pressure cooker's lid, the delicious aroma will be hard to resist. Salmon chowder is also a budget-friendly way to indulge the whole family with just one beautiful piece of salmon.

2 tablespoons butter

1 leek, white and light-green parts only, sliced

3 shallots or 1 small onion, chopped

6 mushrooms, sliced

4 cups vegetable broth, store-bought or homemade (page 222)

1 (6-ounce) salmon fillet, cut into 1-inch chunks

4 medium red potatoes, peeled and cut into ½-inch chunks

2 carrots, cut into ½-inch chunks

1 cup frozen corn kernels (no need to thaw)

1 tablespoon dried dill

1 teaspoon sea salt

1 tablespoon cornstarch

1 cup heavy (whipping) cream or whole milk

1. Select sauté. Add the butter, leek, shallots, and mushrooms and sauté for 3 minutes, or until the shallots are translucent.

2. Add the broth, salmon, potatoes, carrots, corn, dill, and salt.

3. Secure the lid and cook on high pressure for 12 minutes, then allow the pressure to naturally release. Press cancel and remove the lid.

4. Select sauté. Whisk in the cornstarch and cook, whisking, for about 5 minutes to thicken.

5. Whisk in the cream and serve.

STORAGE: Refrigerate in a sealed container for up to 5 days.

INGREDIENT TIP: Frozen salmon can also be used in this recipe. Thaw the fish by placing it in warm water in a plastic bag until you can cut it into chunks.

5 Meatless Mains

Three-Cheese Risotto

SERVES 6
PREP TIME: 10 MINUTES • COOK TIME: 13 MINUTES • TOTAL TIME: 40 MINUTES
PRESSURE RELEASE: NATURAL
ESSENTIAL RECIPE, GLUTEN-FREE, ONE-POT MEAL, UNDER AN HOUR, VEGETARIAN

My mom's family hails from Northern Italy, and I have always watched my mom cook risotto the traditional way on the stove. I must admit I was skeptical when I first heard risotto could be made in an electric pressure cooker, but I am so happy I tried it. This risotto is the ultimate creamy, cheesy treat.

1 tablespoon olive oil

3 shallots, chopped

3 garlic cloves, minced

1 teaspoon herbes de Provence

1 cup Arborio rice

3 cups water or chicken stock, store-bought or homemade (page 223)

⅓ cup grated Parmesan cheese

⅓ cup Asiago cheese

⅓ cup grated white Cheddar cheese

1. Select sauté and let the pot heat up for 2 minutes.

2. Pour the olive oil into the pot, then add the shallots, garlic, and herbes de Provence and sauté for 3 minutes, or until the shallots are translucent.

3. Add the rice and toast it for 1 to 2 minutes. Add the water.

4. Secure the lid and cook on high pressure for 8 minutes, then allow the pressure to naturally release for at least 10 minutes (as the rice will continue cooking during this time). Press cancel.

5. Remove the lid and stir in the three cheeses while the rice is still piping hot. Serve.

STORAGE: Refrigerate in an airtight container for up to 5 days.

INGREDIENT TIP: This recipe only works with white Arborio rice. Lundberg Family Farms is the brand I always buy.

Mushroom Risotto

SERVES 6

PREP TIME: 10 MINUTES • COOK TIME: 13 MINUTES • TOTAL TIME: 40 MINUTES

PRESSURE RELEASE: NATURAL

GLUTEN-FREE, ONE-POT MEAL, UNDER AN HOUR, VEGETARIAN

I have very fond memories of eating mushroom risotto (possibly my favorite dish) sitting in my mother's kitchen. I love that I can now make restaurant-quality risotto in my pressure cooker without standing by the stove and stirring as it cooks. The combination of mushrooms and shallots cooked together in olive oil is unstoppable. You can use one small onion in place of the shallots, but I highly recommend the shallots.

1 tablespoon olive oil

8 ounces baby bella mushrooms, chopped

3 shallots, chopped

3 garlic cloves, minced

1 teaspoon chopped fresh thyme

1 cup Arborio rice

3 cups water or chicken stock, store-bought or homemade (page 223)

½ cup grated Parmesan cheese

1. Select sauté and let the pot heat up for 2 minutes.

2. Pour the olive oil into the pot, then add the mushrooms, shallots, garlic, and thyme. Sauté for 3 minutes, or until the shallots are translucent.

3. Add the rice and toast for 1 to 2 minutes. Add the water.

4. Secure the lid and cook on high pressure for 8 minutes, then allow the pressure to naturally release for at least 10 minutes (the rice will continue cooking during this time). Press cancel.

5. Remove the lid, stir in the Parmesan cheese while the rice is still piping hot, and serve.

STORAGE: Refrigerate in an airtight container for up to 5 days.

INGREDIENT TIP: If you prefer a different mushroom, you can add 8 ounces of your favorite mushroom in place of the baby bellas.

Tomato Risotto

SERVES 6
PREP TIME: 10 MINUTES • COOK TIME: 13 MINUTES • TOTAL TIME: 40 MINUTES
PRESSURE RELEASE: NATURAL
GLUTEN-FREE, ONE-POT MEAL, UNDER AN HOUR, VEGETARIAN

I promise you, if this risotto exists in your house, you will want to eat nothing else. Tomato risotto tastes fresh and filling and is packed with nutty Parmesan cheese. You will love the sweet taste of basil, the savory tomatoes, and the low-maintenance approach to cooking this dish.

1 tablespoon olive oil

3 shallots, chopped

3 garlic cloves, minced

1 teaspoon dried basil

1 cup Arborio rice

2 cups water or chicken stock, store-bought or homemade (page 223)

1 (14.5-ounce) can diced tomatoes

½ cup grated Parmesan cheese

1. Select sauté and let the pot heat up for 2 minutes.

2. Pour the olive oil into the pot, then add the shallots, garlic, and dried basil. Sauté for 3 minutes, or until the shallots are translucent.

3. Add the rice and toast for 1 to 2 minutes. Add the water and tomatoes.

4. Secure the lid and cook on high pressure for 8 minutes, then allow the pressure to naturally release. Press cancel.

5. Remove the lid, stir in the Parmesan cheese while the rice is still piping hot, and serve.

STORAGE: Refrigerate in an airtight container for up to 5 days.

INGREDIENT TIP: You can use fresh tomatoes in place of canned in this recipe, but if you use canned, I recommend Red Gold brand.

Pasta with Mushroom-Tarragon Sauce

SERVES 6

PREP TIME: 10 MINUTES • COOK TIME: 5 MINUTES • TOTAL TIME: 30 MINUTES

PRESSURE RELEASE: QUICK

ONE-POT MEAL, UNDER AN HOUR, VEGETARIAN

The creamy mushroom and herb–infused sauce makes this pasta a family-pleasing dinner option for any night of the week, and it is great for leftovers, too. Once you try it, you'll be hooked, because it is delicious enough to serve to company but also effortless to prepare. This is a one-pot meal that will leave you with literally only one pot to wash once it's done.

4 cups water

12 ounces button mushrooms, sliced

2 tablespoons olive oil

1 shallot, chopped

2 teaspoons chopped fresh tarragon

12 ounces spaghetti or linguine, broken in half

¼ cup shredded mozzarella cheese

½ cup heavy (whipping) cream or half-and-half

½ cup grated Parmesan cheese

1 tablespoon grated lemon zest

1. In the inner pot, combine the water, mushrooms, oil, shallot, and tarragon.

2. Add the spaghetti to the pot, pushing it down to make sure it is covered entirely with liquid.

3. Secure the lid and cook on high pressure for 5 minutes, then quick release the pressure and remove the lid. Press cancel.

4. Stir in the mozzarella and cream while the pasta is still piping hot. Don't worry about excess liquid. It will thicken in a few minutes.

5. After 5 minutes, once the pasta has been able to thicken with the cheese, stir in the Parmesan and top with the lemon zest. Serve.

STORAGE: Refrigerate in an airtight container for up to 5 days.

INGREDIENT TIP: You can make this recipe with a generous ½ teaspoon of dried tarragon in place of the fresh tarragon.

Creamy Tortellini with Peas

SERVES 6

PREP TIME: 10 MINUTES • COOK TIME: 5 MINUTES • TOTAL TIME: 25 MINUTES

PRESSURE RELEASE: QUICK

ONE-POT MEAL, UNDER 30 MINUTES, VEGETARIAN

Creamy pasta with peas is a classic dinner in the Midwest. This comforting dish comes together very quickly, and the lovely contrast of bright green peas in a cheesy white sauce is like spring on a plate.

2 cups water

2 cups chicken stock, store-bought or homemade (page 223)

12 ounces dried tortellini

1 (12-ounce) bag frozen peas (no need to thaw)

1 tablespoon olive oil

3 garlic cloves, minced

1 cup shredded mozzarella cheese

½ cup grated Parmesan cheese

¼ cup half-and-half or whole milk

1. In the inner pot, combine the water, chicken stock, tortellini, peas, olive oil, and garlic. Stir and make sure the pasta is completely submerged in the liquid.

2. Secure the lid and cook on high pressure for 5 minutes, then quick release the pressure and remove the lid. Press cancel.

3. Stir in the mozzarella, Parmesan, and half-and-half while the tortellini are still piping hot until the cheeses are completely melted. Serve.

STORAGE: Refrigerate in an airtight container for up to 5 days.

INGREDIENT TIP: This recipe is for dried tortellini. If you're cooking with fresh tortellini, cook it for half the time listed on the pasta package—a general rule for cooking pasta in an electric pressure cooker.

Angel Hair with Parmesan

SERVES 4 TO 6
PREP TIME: 5 MINUTES • COOK TIME: 3 MINUTES • TOTAL TIME: 20 MINUTES
PRESSURE RELEASE: QUICK
ONE-POT MEAL, UNDER 30 MINUTES, VEGETARIAN

One of my kids' favorite meals is this simple, 5-ingredient pasta decked out with lots of Parmesan cheese on top. It is appropriate for dinner any night of the week. If you have any leftovers, this meal makes great lunch the following day.

1 tablespoon olive oil

4 cups water

2 tablespoons freshly squeezed lemon juice

1 garlic clove, minced

12 ounces angel hair pasta, broken in half

8 ounces Parmesan cheese, grated

1. Coat the bottom of the inner pot with the olive oil. Add the water, lemon juice, and garlic. Add the pasta to the pot and stir to make sure it is submerged in the water.

2. Secure the lid and cook on high pressure for 3 minutes, then quick release the pressure and remove the lid. Press cancel.

3. Let the pasta cool for about 5 minutes. Stir in the Parmesan cheese until well coated and serve.

STORAGE: Refrigerate in an airtight container for up to 5 days.

MENU PLANNING TIP: Mushroom Bourguignon (page 118) tastes great on top of this angel hair pasta.

Vegetable Lasagna

SERVES 4
PREP TIME: 10 MINUTES • COOK TIME: 24 MINUTES • TOTAL TIME: 50 MINUTES
PRESSURE RELEASE: NATURAL
ONE-POT MEAL, UNDER AN HOUR, VEGETARIAN

Once you learn how to make lasagna in your electric pressure cooker, you may never go back to making it in the oven. You can easily switch this recipe up by using whatever vegetables you have on hand. This dish uses no-boil noodles, is packed with vegetables, and is an incredibly comforting vegetarian dinner recipe that satisfies everyone's taste buds.

1 tablespoon olive oil

12 ounces white mushrooms, sliced

1 cup ricotta cheese

1 cup grated Parmesan cheese

1 large egg

1 teaspoon Italian seasoning

2 cups Marinara Sauce (page 232)

6 no-boil lasagna noodles, broken up

4 cups chopped stemmed fresh spinach or baby spinach

1 cup water

½ cup shredded mozzarella cheese

1. Select sauté and let the pot heat up for 2 minutes.

2. Pour the olive oil into the pot, then add the mushrooms and sauté for 3 to 4 minutes, until they are softened. Press cancel. Remove the mushrooms and set aside.

3. Rinse out the inner pot and scrape off any bits of food stuck on the bottom. Return the pot to the pressure cooker.

4. In a medium bowl, mix the ricotta, Parmesan, egg, and Italian seasoning.

5. Spread half the marinara sauce in the bottom of a 7-inch springform pan. Arrange half of the broken lasagna noodles in a single layer over the sauce, pushing them down into the sauce so that they are covered. Spread on half of the cheese mixture, followed by half the spinach and half the mushrooms.

6. Add the remaining sauce and lasagna noodles, again pressing the noodles down so that they are covered in sauce. Then add the remaining cheese mixture, spinach, and mushrooms.

7. Pour the water into the pot and insert a trivet or a silicone sling (if you don't have a sling or a trivet with handles, fashion a foil sling and place it on the trivet). Place the springform pan on top.

8. Secure the lid and cook on high pressure for 20 minutes, then allow the pressure to naturally release. Press cancel.

9. Remove the lid and carefully lift the springform pan out of the pot. Don't worry if the lasagna looks a little watery on top. It will thicken in a few minutes.

10. Top with the mozzarella and serve.

STORAGE: Refrigerate in an airtight container for up to 5 days.

SWITCH IT UP: You can make this lasagna with any vegetables you have available. Broccoli, tomatoes, summer squash, and eggplant would taste great.

Gnocchi Lasagna

SERVES 4
PREP TIME: 10 MINUTES • COOK TIME: 20 MINUTES • TOTAL TIME: 50 MINUTES
PRESSURE RELEASE: NATURAL
ONE-POT MEAL, UNDER AN HOUR, VEGETARIAN

Pressure cooker gnocchi lasagna is mind-blowingly good because the gnocchi absorb the flavor from the sauce that they are cooked in. Replacing traditional lasagna noodles with gnocchi creates a casserole-like meal rather than distinct layers, but it still looks spectacular. I have also included a gluten-free variation (see tip) using frozen cauliflower gnocchi.

1 cup ricotta cheese

1 cup grated
Parmesan cheese

1 large egg

1 teaspoon Italian seasoning

2 cups Marinara Sauce
(page 232)

1 (16-ounce) container fresh
or frozen gnocchi

1 cup water

½ cup shredded
mozzarella cheese

1. In a medium bowl, combine the ricotta, Parmesan, egg, and Italian seasoning until well mixed.

2. Line the bottom of a 7-inch springform pan with half the marinara sauce. Arrange one layer of gnocchi in the pan and spread half of the ricotta cheese mixture over the gnocchi.

3. Add the remaining sauce and gnocchi, making sure the gnocchi are covered in sauce. Top with the remaining ricotta mixture.

4. Pour the water into the inner pot and insert a trivet or a silicone sling (if you don't have a sling or a trivet with handles, fashion a foil sling and place it on the trivet). Place the springform pan on top.

5. Secure the lid and cook on high pressure for 20 minutes, then allow the pressure to naturally release. Press cancel.

6. Remove the lid and carefully lift the pan out of the pot. Don't worry if the lasagna looks a little watery on top. It will thicken in a few minutes.

7. Top with the mozzarella and serve.

STORAGE: Refrigerate in an airtight container for up to 5 days.

SWITCH IT UP: This recipe also works with frozen cauliflower gnocchi. Replace the gnocchi with cauliflower gnocchi in the same amount.

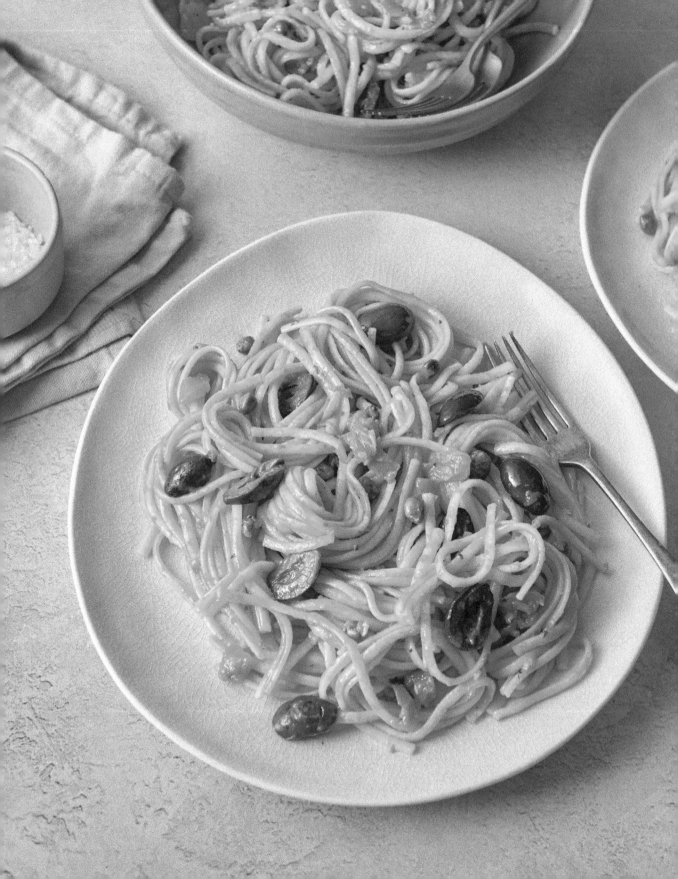

Linguine Puttanesca

SERVES 4 TO 6
PREP TIME: 5 MINUTES • COOK TIME: 5 MINUTES • TOTAL TIME: 20 MINUTES
PRESSURE RELEASE: QUICK
ONE-POT MEAL, UNDER 30 MINUTES, VEGAN

This linguine dish is incredibly flavorful thanks to the inclusion of kalamata olives and capers, two ingredients you might already have in your pantry. You can whip up this dish in the pressure cooker in a matter of minutes, and your meal will be Italian-restaurant quality. Anchovies add depth and satisfying saltiness to the dish, so even if they are not a favorite ingredient, I encourage you to try them. You might be surprised at the result.

3 tablespoons olive oil

4 cups water

1 (28-ounce) can crushed tomatoes

½ cup halved pitted kalamata olives

2 tablespoons tomato paste

4 garlic cloves, minced

1 tablespoon brine from the olive jar

1½ teaspoons capers

1 teaspoon brine from the caper jar

1 teaspoon Italian seasoning

1 teaspoon anchovy paste (optional)

½ teaspoon red pepper flakes

16 ounces linguine, broken in half

1. Coat the bottom of the inner pot with the olive oil. Add the water, tomatoes, olives, tomato paste, garlic, olive brine, capers, caper brine, Italian seasoning, anchovy paste (if using), and red pepper flakes.

2. Add the linguine to the pot and stir the ingredients together, ensuring the pasta is covered in liquid.

3. Secure the lid and cook on high pressure for 5 minutes, then quick release the pressure and remove the lid. Press cancel.

4. Don't worry if the pasta looks runny; let it sit for a few minutes before serving. It will thicken once it cools down. Serve.

STORAGE: Refrigerate in an airtight container for up to 5 days.

INGREDIENT TIP: If you don't have linguine, you can also use spaghetti. Or if you want to choose another pasta shape, go for the thinner or smaller shapes as they work best in the electric pressure cooker.

Greek-Inspired Orzo with Tomatoes and Olives

SERVES 4 TO 6

PREP TIME: 10 MINUTES • COOK TIME: 5 MINUTES • TOTAL TIME: 25 MINUTES

PRESSURE RELEASE: QUICK

ONE-POT MEAL, UNDER 30 MINUTES, VEGETARIAN

With a pressure-cooking time of 3 minutes and ingredients that you might already have in your cupboard, this Mediterranean-influenced meal couldn't be easier. This dish is delicious served hot or cold, making it a refreshing lunch or dinner recipe to enjoy year-round. Add your favorite Greek toppings—like feta cheese and fresh dill—to pump up the flavor.

2 tablespoons olive oil

½ onion, chopped

2 garlic cloves, minced

2 teaspoons oregano

1 teaspoon Greek seasoning

3½ cups water

16 ounces orzo

1 (14.5-ounce) can diced tomatoes

¼ cup sliced pitted kalamata olives, plus 2 tablespoons for serving

2 tablespoons brine from the olive jar

2 tablespoons crumbled feta cheese, for serving (optional)

2 tablespoons chopped fresh dill, for serving (optional)

1. Select sauté and let the pot heat up for 2 minutes.

2. Add the olive oil, onion, garlic, oregano, and Greek seasoning and sauté for 2 minutes, or until the onions are translucent.

3. Add the water, orzo, tomatoes, ¼ cup kalamata olives, and olive brine, making sure that the pasta is completely submerged in the water.

4. Secure the lid and cook on high pressure for 3 minutes, then quick release the pressure and remove the lid. Press cancel.

5. Serve topped with the 2 tablespoons kalamata olives. If desired, sprinkle with feta cheese and dill.

STORAGE: Refrigerate in an airtight container for up to 5 days.

SWITCH IT UP: This dish can be made with any pasta shape you like. If you choose to use another shape, remember to use enough water to submerge the pasta completely.

Macaroni and Cheese

SERVES 4 TO 6
PREP TIME: 5 MINUTES • COOK TIME: 5 MINUTES • TOTAL TIME: 20 MINUTES
PRESSURE RELEASE: QUICK
ONE-POT MEAL, UNDER 30 MINUTES, VEGETARIAN

Preparing homemade macaroni and cheese in the electric pressure cooker has several benefits. It is healthier, quicker, and tastes better than the boxed version. Your kids will never ask for "powdered cheese" macaroni again after trying this melty, gooey, and cheesy meal. It might become your favorite comfort food, as well.

4 cups water

16 ounces elbow macaroni

2 tablespoons butter

1 teaspoon mustard powder

3 cups shredded Cheddar cheese

½ cup half-and-half or whole milk

1. In the inner pot, combine the water, macaroni, butter, and mustard powder.

2. Secure the lid and cook on high pressure for 5 minutes, then quick release the pressure and remove the lid.

3. Stir in the Cheddar cheese and half-and-half while the noodles are still piping hot, until the consistency is smooth and velvety. Serve.

STORAGE: Refrigerate in an airtight container for up to 5 days.

SWITCH IT UP: You don't have to stick with Cheddar here: You can make macaroni and cheese with your favorite cheese or combination of cheeses.

Tomato-Basil Macaroni and Cheese

SERVES 4 TO 6
PREP TIME: 5 MINUTES • COOK TIME: 5 MINUTES • TOTAL TIME: 20 MINUTES
PRESSURE RELEASE: QUICK
ONE-POT MEAL, UNDER 30 MINUTES, VEGETARIAN

When tomatoes start to pop up in my garden midsummer, I put them in every recipe I can think of. This dressed-up mac and cheese is bright, fresh, and colorful. It is appropriate for lunch or dinner during the summer, and you won't need to heat up your kitchen to make it. This meal is a tasty way to liven up your dinner rotation.

4 cups water

16 ounces elbow macaroni

2 cups halved grape tomatoes

2 tablespoons butter

1½ cups shredded mozzarella cheese

1½ cups shredded Cheddar cheese

½ cup half-and-half or whole milk

¼ cup chopped fresh basil

1. In the inner pot, combine the water, macaroni, tomatoes, and butter.

2. Secure the lid and cook on high pressure for 5 minutes, then quick release the pressure and remove the lid. Press cancel.

3. Add the mozzarella, Cheddar, and half-and-half while the noodles are still piping hot, stirring to combine.

4. Stir in the basil and serve.

STORAGE: Refrigerate in an airtight container for up to 5 days.

INGREDIENT TIP: If you don't have fresh tomatoes, use 1 (14.5-ounce) can of diced tomatoes.

Creamy Quinoa Veggie Casserole

SERVES 4
PREP TIME: 5 MINUTES • COOK TIME: 1 MINUTE • TOTAL TIME: 20 MINUTES
PRESSURE RELEASE: NATURAL
GLUTEN-FREE, ONE-POT MEAL, UNDER 30 MINUTES, VEGETARIAN

When I learned how to cook quick casseroles in my electric pressure cooker, it was a game-changer. This light, flavorful vegetarian casserole is a good showcase for how quick and easy cooking casseroles can be with the pressure cooker. Feel free to improvise with this recipe and add whatever leftovers you have in the fridge.

2 cups water

2 cups chopped broccoli

1 (12-ounce) bag frozen mixed vegetables (no need to thaw)

1 cup quinoa

½ cup chopped onion

1 tablespoon butter

1 garlic clove, minced

1 tablespoon Greek seasoning

1 cup shredded Cheddar cheese

1 cup shredded Monterey Jack cheese

1. In the inner pot, combine the water, broccoli, mixed vegetables, quinoa, onion, butter, garlic, and Greek seasoning.

2. Secure the lid and cook on high pressure for 1 minute. Allow the pressure to naturally release for 5 minutes, then quick release the remaining pressure and remove the lid. Press cancel.

3. Stir in the Cheddar and Monterey Jack cheeses while the quinoa and vegetables are piping hot. Serve.

STORAGE: Refrigerate in an airtight container for up to 5 days.

SWITCH IT UP: This casserole can be a blank slate, so add your favorite seasonings instead of the Greek seasoning to make it your own.

Mushroom Bourguignon

SERVES 4
PREP TIME: 10 MINUTES • COOK TIME: 12 MINUTES • TOTAL TIME: 25 MINUTES
PRESSURE RELEASE: QUICK
DAIRY-FREE, GLUTEN-FREE, ONE-POT MEAL, UNDER 30 MINUTES, VEGAN

I enjoy serving my family plant-based foods at least once a week. This Mushroom Bourguignon is the perfect dish for a "meatless Monday" or any night when you're craving a tasty, hearty, filling meal.

2 tablespoons olive oil

1 cup frozen pearl onions (no need to thaw)

3 shallots, chopped

2 cups vegetable broth, store-bought or homemade (page 222)

1 cup dry red wine

2 pounds mushrooms, sliced

4 medium carrots, cut into 1-inch chunks

1 tablespoon tomato paste

2 teaspoons herbes de Provence

1 tablespoon cornstarch

1. Select sauté and let the pot heat up for 2 minutes.

2. Add the olive oil, pearl onions, and shallots and sauté for 2 minutes, until the onions are translucent.

3. Add the broth, red wine, mushrooms, carrots, tomato paste, and herbes de Provence.

4. Secure the lid and cook on high pressure for 5 minutes, then quick release the pressure and remove the lid. Press cancel.

5. Select sauté. Whisk the cornstarch into the pot and whisk for 5 minutes to thicken the stew. Serve.

STORAGE: Refrigerate in an airtight container for up to 5 days.

MENU PLANNING TIP: I enjoy this stew over Parmesan Polenta (page 71), Farro (page 67), or linguine pasta.

Vegan Black Bean Burrito Bowls

SERVES 6
PREP TIME: 5 MINUTES • COOK TIME: 12 MINUTES • TOTAL TIME: 30 MINUTES
PRESSURE RELEASE: QUICK
GLUTEN-FREE, ONE-POT MEAL, UNDER AN HOUR, VEGAN

My family has embraced burrito bowls, where rice and beans are paired with glorious Southwestern toppings, as a favorite meal choice. This pressure-cooker version features salsa, corn, beans, and seasonings cooked right into the rice. I love adding shredded lettuce, avocado, cheese, and lime juice on top of mine and enjoy serving this dish at parties because everyone can add their favorite toppings.

1 (15-ounce) can black beans, drained and rinsed, or 1½ cups Black Beans (page 48)

1¾ cups water

1 cup raw white rice, rinsed

1 cup frozen corn kernels (no need to thaw)

1 cup store-bought salsa

½ onion, chopped

1 teaspoon ground cumin

1 teaspoon chili powder

1 teaspoon sea salt

Optional toppings

½ cup shredded Cotija cheese

¼ cup chopped tomato

½ cup chopped lettuce

1 teaspoon freshly squeezed lime juice

2 tablespoons sour cream

½ cup Garden Salsa (page 231)

1. In the inner pot, combine the black beans, water, rice, corn, salsa, onion, cumin, chili powder, and salt.

2. Secure the lid and cook on high pressure for 12 minutes, then quick release the pressure and remove the lid. Press cancel.

3. Mix the rice mixture with a wooden spoon or spatula. Scoop the rice into individual bowls and let each person add their desired toppings.

MENU PLANNING TIP: The Basic Salsa Pulled Pork (page 167) would make a great additional topping for these burrito bowls.

Refried Bean Tacos with Cilantro Slaw

SERVES 4 TO 6
PREP TIME: 5 MINUTES • COOK TIME: 35 MINUTES • TOTAL TIME: 1 HOUR
5 MINUTES
▶ **PRESSURE RELEASE:** NATURAL
GLUTEN-FREE, ONE-POT MEAL, VEGETARIAN, WORTH THE WAIT

This recipe is a unique vegetarian dinner that is sure to satisfy. The creamy homemade refried beans taste delicious with the flavorful, fresh, and crunchy cilantro slaw. Your family will get loads of plant-based protein from this meal, and they won't miss the meat at all.

For the refried beans

1 medium onion, chopped

8 cups water

2 cups dried pinto beans

1 garlic clove, minced

1 tablespoon freshly squeezed lime juice

1 tablespoon ground cumin

2 teaspoons sea salt

For the cilantro dressing

½ cup chopped fresh cilantro

½ cup chopped avocado

¼ cup yogurt

1 tablespoon freshly squeezed lime juice

1 teaspoon distilled white vinegar

¼ teaspoon ground cumin

To make the refried beans

1. In the inner pot, combine the onion, water, beans, garlic, lime juice, cumin, and salt.

2. Secure the lid and select the "bean/chili" mode, or cook on high pressure for 30 minutes. Allow the pressure to naturally release. Press cancel and open the lid.

To make the cilantro dressing

3. While the beans are cooking, in a blender or food processor, puree the cilantro, avocado, yogurt, lime juice, vinegar, and cumin until smooth.

To make the cilantro slaw

4. In a medium bowl. combine the coleslaw mix, bell pepper, corn, carrot, cilantro, and scallions and toss to mix. Add the dressing and toss until the vegetables are well coated. Refrigerate and let the slaw marinate for at least 30 minutes before eating.

For the cilantro slaw

1 (16-ounce) bag
coleslaw mix

1 red, yellow, or orange bell
pepper, chopped

1 cup fresh or thawed frozen
corn kernels

1 carrot, chopped

1 to 3 cilantro
sprigs, chopped

2 scallions, chopped

For serving

3 tablespoons vegetable oil

Soft 6- or 8-inch flour
tortillas, for serving

To serve

5. Drain the beans and return them to the inner pot. Select sauté. Add the vegetable oil and sauté the beans for 5 minutes while smashing them with a spatula or wooden spoon.

6. Spread the refried beans onto a warmed tortilla, top with cilantro slaw, and serve.

SWITCH IT UP: You could use corn tortillas in place of the flour tortillas.

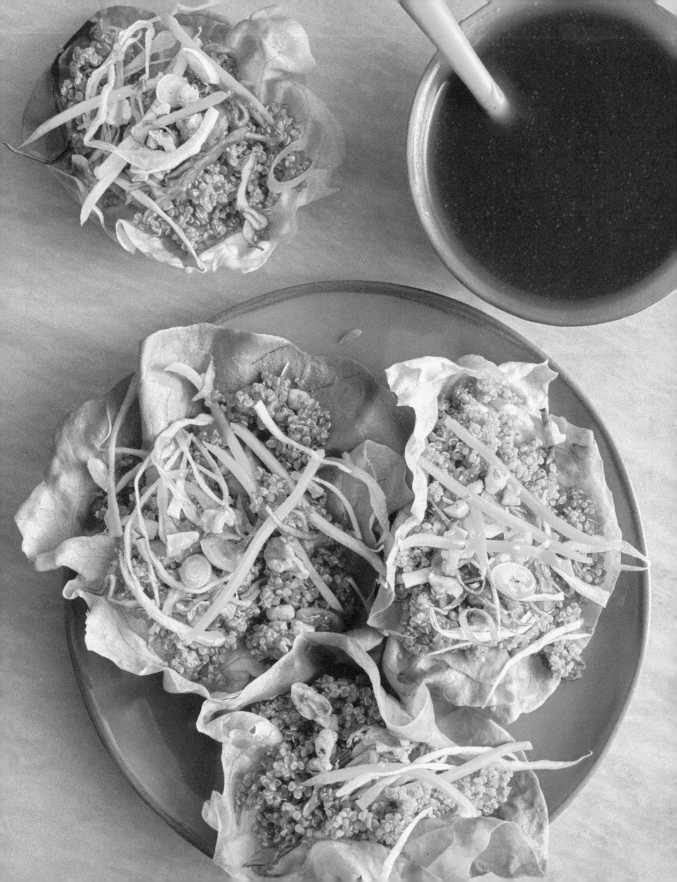

Chinese Five-Spice Quinoa Lettuce Wraps

SERVES 4 TO 6
PREP TIME: 10 MINUTES • COOK TIME: 6 MINUTES • TOTAL TIME: 30 MINUTES
PRESSURE RELEASE: NATURAL
DAIRY-FREE, ONE-POT MEAL, UNDER AN HOUR, VEGAN

Lettuce wraps might seem like a lighter meal, especially this vegan version, but my guess is that this dish will satisfy everyone at your table. The quinoa is packed with flavor because it is cooked in Chinese five-spice powder, brown sugar, garlic, and soy sauce. The lettuce wraps are topped with toasty walnuts, crunchy carrots, and cabbage and finished off with sweet hoisin sauce. This is a perfect dinner or appetizer to serve on a hot night when you don't want to heat up the house by turning on the stove.

2 cups water

1 cup quinoa

2 garlic cloves, minced

1 tablespoon soy sauce

1 tablespoon light
brown sugar

1 teaspoon Chinese
five-spice powder

½ cup chopped walnuts

1 head butter lettuce,
separated into leaves,
washed and dried

2 carrots, cut
into matchsticks

1 cup shredded cabbage

¼ cup chopped scallions

¼ cup hoisin sauce

1. In the inner pot, combine the water, quinoa, garlic, soy sauce, brown sugar, and Chinese five-spice powder.

2. Secure the lid and cook on high pressure for 1 minute, then allow the pressure to naturally release. Press cancel.

3. Remove the lid and transfer the quinoa to a bowl. Select sauté and add the walnuts in a single layer to the inner pot. Toast the walnuts for 5 minutes and chop.

4. Scoop the quinoa into the lettuce leaves and top with the carrots, cabbage, scallions, and toasted walnuts. Drizzle with the hoisin sauce and serve.

INGREDIENT TIP: To make these gluten-free, substitute tamari for the soy sauce.

Red Lentil Coconut Curry

SERVES 6
PREP TIME: 5 MINUTES • COOK TIME: 8 MINUTES • TOTAL TIME: 35 MINUTES
PRESSURE RELEASE: NATURAL
GLUTEN-FREE, ONE-POT MEAL, UNDER AN HOUR, VEGAN

This simple lentil coconut curry is a great recipe to try if you're looking to dive into the curry world. The combination of coconut milk and sweet tomatoes is marvelous with spicy curry flavoring. The addition of coconut milk makes this a kid-friendly meal. My youngest son loves this recipe and is excited every time I make it.

1 (15-ounce) can crushed tomatoes

1 (15-ounce) can full-fat coconut milk

1 cup water

1 cup red lentils

3 carrots, cut into 1-inch chunks

1 tablespoon curry powder

1 tablespoon freshly squeezed lime juice

1 teaspoon ground ginger

Sticky Rice (page 68), for serving

Chopped fresh cilantro, for garnish (optional)

1. In the inner pot, combine the tomatoes, coconut milk, water, lentils, carrots, curry powder, lime juice, and ginger.

2. Secure the lid and cook on high pressure for 8 minutes, then allow the pressure to naturally release for at least 10 minutes (as the lentils will continue cooking during this time). Remove the lid and press cancel.

3. Serve over rice and garnish with cilantro (if using).

STORAGE: Refrigerate in an airtight container for up to 5 days or freeze up to 2 months.

INGREDIENT TIP: Brown lentils will also work in this recipe.

Jambalaya-Stuffed Peppers

SERVES 6
PREP TIME: 10 MINUTES • COOK TIME: 10 MINUTES • TOTAL TIME: 50 MINUTES
PRESSURE RELEASE: NATURAL
GLUTEN-FREE, ONE-POT MEAL, UNDER AN HOUR, VEGETARIAN

Electric pressure cookers make the most delicious stuffed peppers, hands down. Using jambalaya instead of plain cooked rice creates a flavor-packed vegetarian meal option that only requires a few extra ingredients. These peppers have savory Cajun seasoning, sweet pineapple, zesty tomato sauce, and melty cheese. You can also omit the cheese and make this recipe vegan.

1 cup raw long-grain white rice

3 cups water, divided

½ teaspoon sea salt

1 cup canned tomato sauce

½ cup shredded Monterey Jack cheese

¼ cup finely diced thawed frozen pineapple chunks

2 tablespoons finely chopped onion

2 tablespoons finely chopped celery

1 teaspoon Cajun seasoning

6 green bell peppers

1. In the inner pot, combine the rice, 2 cups water, and salt.

2. Secure the lid and select the "rice" mode, or cook on high pressure for 5 minutes. Allow the pressure to naturally release for at least 10 minutes (as the rice will continue cooking during this time). Press cancel and remove the lid.

3. Transfer the rice to a medium bowl and stir in the tomato sauce, Monterey Jack, pineapple, onion, celery, and Cajun seasoning until well combined.

4. Cut the tops off the peppers, remove the seeds, and evenly divide the rice mixture among them.

5. Rinse out the inner pot and return to the pressure cooker. Pour 1 cup water into the pot and insert the trivet. Set the stuffed peppers on the trivet.

6. Secure the lid and cook on high pressure for 5 minutes, then quick release the pressure and remove the lid. Press cancel.

7. Remove the peppers and serve.

> **INGREDIENT TIP:** This recipe will work with all kinds of cooked rice or grains. You can use cooked quinoa, farro, or brown rice.

Peanut Noodles

SERVES 4 TO 6
PREP TIME: 10 MINUTES • COOK TIME: 5 MINUTES • TOTAL TIME: 25 MINUTES
PRESSURE RELEASE: QUICK
DAIRY-FREE, ONE-POT MEAL, UNDER 30 MINUTES, VEGAN

Thai-style peanut noodles is one of my favorite dishes and was the first take-out dish that I learned how to make at home. My oldest son is very partial to these noodles, so for me the ingredients here are pantry staples. I always have toasted sesame oil, ginger, hoisin sauce, and rice vinegar on hand, and with the electric pressure cooker, I can make this dish in a flash.

⅔ cup peanut butter

6 tablespoons soy sauce

¼ cup packed light brown sugar

2 tablespoons hoisin sauce

2 tablespoons rice vinegar

2 tablespoons freshly squeezed lime juice

2 garlic cloves, minced

1 tablespoon sesame oil

1 teaspoon ground ginger

3 cups water

8 ounces spaghetti, broken in half

1 (12-ounce) bag frozen stir-fry vegetables (or chopped fresh vegetables)

½ cup crushed peanuts, for serving

1. Select sauté. Add the peanut butter, soy sauce, brown sugar, hoisin, vinegar, lime juice, garlic, sesame oil, and ginger. Whisk the ingredients together and cook until melted and heated through. Press cancel.

2. Stir the water into the sauce and add the spaghetti, making sure it is submerged. Place the frozen vegetables into the vegetable steamer and add it to the pot.

3. Secure the lid and cook on high pressure for 5 minutes, then quick release the pressure and remove the lid. Press cancel.

4. Tip the vegetables out of the steamer basket into a bowl. Add the noodles and sauce and stir to combine.

5. Serve topped with the crushed peanuts.

STORAGE: Refrigerate in an airtight container for up to 5 days.

SWITCH IT UP: You can make this meal gluten-free by replacing the spaghetti with Thai rice noodles and replacing the soy sauce with tamari sauce.

Coconut-Curry Rice with Cauliflower

SERVES 4 TO 6
PREP TIME: 10 MINUTES • **COOK TIME:** 14 MINUTES • **TOTAL TIME:** 35 MINUTES
PRESSURE RELEASE: NATURAL
DAIRY-FREE, GLUTEN-FREE, ONE-POT MEAL, UNDER AN HOUR, VEGETARIAN

You will love the way the cauliflower soaks up all the flavors in this easy one-pot meal. I first realized that I enjoyed coconut curry several years ago in a Thai restaurant, but I never thought I could make it at home. Once I started seeing Thai ingredients popping up in my local grocery stores, I became inspired and started trying different recipes. Here's how to make my favorite version.

3 cups water

2 cups jasmine rice

2 cups cauliflower florets

1 (15-ounce) can full-fat coconut milk

1 (12-ounce) bag frozen carrots and peas (no need to thaw)

1 tablespoon sesame oil

1 shallot or ½ small onion, chopped

1 garlic clove, minced

2 tablespoons curry powder

1 large egg, lightly beaten

½ cup crushed peanuts

¼ cup chopped scallions, green part only

1. In the inner pot, combine the water, rice, cauliflower, coconut milk, frozen vegetables, sesame oil, shallot, garlic, and curry powder.

2. Secure the lid and select the "rice" mode, or cook on high pressure for 12 minutes. Allow the pressure to naturally release for at least 10 minutes (as the rice will continue cooking during that time). Press cancel.

3. Remove the lid and transfer the rice to a serving bowl.

4. Select sauté and let the pot heat up for 2 minutes. Add the egg to the pot and scramble. Mix the scrambled egg into the rice.

5. Serve topped with peanuts and scallion greens.

STORAGE: Refrigerate in an airtight container for up to 5 days.

INGREDIENT TIP: This recipe works best with jasmine and long-grain Thai rice.

Almond and Thai Basil Fried Rice

SERVES 4 TO 6
PREP TIME: 10 MINUTES • COOK TIME: 16 MINUTES • TOTAL TIME: 35 MINUTES
PRESSURE RELEASE: NATURAL
DAIRY-FREE, ONE-POT MEAL, UNDER AN HOUR, VEGETARIAN

The combination of almond and Thai basil has become one of my favorite flavor profiles over the years. It all started when I ordered Thai basil noodles from a local restaurant and then experimented with Thai basil in different dishes at home. Fried rice is an easy one-pot dinner that tastes nutty and sweet with hints of basil—a perfect dish to make when you want to use freshly grown herbs.

1 tablespoon sesame oil

1 shallot or ½ small onion, chopped

1 garlic clove, minced

3 tablespoons almond butter

2 tablespoons fresh Thai basil

1 tablespoon freshly squeezed lime juice

1 tablespoon soy sauce

2 teaspoons canned full-fat coconut milk

3 cups water

2 cups jasmine rice

1 (12-ounce) bag frozen carrots and peas (no need to thaw)

1 large egg, lightly beaten

1. Select sauté and let the pot heat up for 2 minutes.

2. Add the sesame oil, shallot, and garlic and sauté for 2 minutes, or until the shallot is translucent.

3. Add the almond butter, basil, lime juice, soy sauce, and coconut milk. Whisk together until well combined, then add the water, rice, and frozen vegetables.

4. Secure the lid and cook on high pressure for 12 minutes, then allow the pressure to naturally release for at least 10 minutes (as the rice will continue cooking during this time). Press cancel.

5. Remove the lid and transfer the rice to a serving bowl.

6. Select sauté and let the pot heat up for 2 minutes. Add the egg to the pot and scramble. Mix the scrambled egg into the rice and serve.

INGREDIENT TIP: This recipe works best with jasmine and long-grain Thai rice.

Double-Ginger Lo Mein

SERVES 6
PREP TIME: 10 MINUTES • COOK TIME: 5 MINUTES • TOTAL TIME: 25 MINUTES
PRESSURE RELEASE: QUICK
DAIRY-FREE, ONE-POT MEAL, UNDER 30 MINUTES, VEGAN

Ginger is one of my favorite spices, and I love adding lots of it to Asian-inspired meals. This recipe is infused with ginger in two ways: The liquid used to cook the noodles and make the sauce includes both brewed ginger tea and ground ginger. The noodles and the vegetables cook together in the pot, and the whole meal takes less than 30 minutes.

2 cups water

1 cup brewed ginger tea

3 tablespoons soy sauce

2 tablespoons light brown sugar

1 tablespoon sesame oil

2 garlic cloves, minced

1 teaspoon ground ginger

8 ounces linguine or spaghetti, broken in half

1 (12-ounce) bag frozen stir-fry vegetables (or chopped fresh vegetables)

¼ cup peanuts

2 tablespoons chopped scallions

1 tablespoon sesame seeds

1. In the inner pot, combine the water, ginger tea, soy sauce, brown sugar, sesame oil, garlic, and ginger. Add the pasta, making sure that it is submerged.

2. Place the vegetables in a vegetable steamer and set it on top of the noodles.

3. Secure the lid and cook on high pressure for 5 minutes, then quick release the pressure and remove the lid. Press cancel.

4. Transfer the vegetables to a bowl. Tip in the noodles and sauce and stir together. Serve topped with the peanuts, scallions, and sesame seeds.

STORAGE: Refrigerate in an airtight container for up to 5 days.

Southwestern Veggie Egg Roll in a Bowl

SERVES 4
PREP TIME: 5 MINUTES • COOK TIME: 0 MINUTES • TOTAL TIME: 15 MINUTES
PRESSURE RELEASE: QUICK
DAIRY-FREE, GLUTEN-FREE, ONE-POT MEAL, UNDER 30 MINUTES, VEGAN

Filled with vegetables, black beans, and an irresistible blend of spices, this Southwestern-inspired bowl is one of my favorite healthy meals to whip up for a quick lunch.

2 (16-ounce) packages coleslaw mix, divided

1 cup frozen corn kernels (no need to thaw)

½ cup cooked black beans, canned or homemade (page 48)

½ cup chopped tomatoes

⅓ cup chopped scallions, green parts only

1 bell pepper, any color, chopped

1 tablespoon vegetable oil

1 teaspoon chili powder

1 teaspoon ground cumin

1 teaspoon dried oregano

1 teaspoon garlic powder

Optional toppings

1 avocado, chopped

¼ cup chopped fresh cilantro

2 tablespoons taco sauce

¼ cup sour cream

1. In the inner pot, combine one bag of coleslaw, the corn, beans, tomatoes, scallion greens, bell pepper, vegetable oil, chili powder, cumin, oregano, and garlic powder.

2. Secure the lid and cook for 0 minutes, then quick release the pressure and remove the lid. Press cancel.

3. Stir in the second bag of coleslaw mix. Serve with any of the toppings you would like.

INGREDIENT TIP: You can use a packet of taco seasoning instead of the seasonings listed.

Smoky Portobello Mushroom Burgers

SERVES 4
PREP TIME: 5 MINUTES • COOK TIME: 0 MINUTES • TOTAL TIME: 15 MINUTES
PRESSURE RELEASE: QUICK
DAIRY-FREE, ONE-POT MEAL, UNDER 30 MINUTES, VEGAN

Instead of buying processed vegetarian burgers, I love to make "burgers" from big, meaty mushrooms. I happen to love portobello mushrooms, and they take the place of beef nicely in a bun with all those glorious burger toppings! These electric pressure cooker mushroom burgers turn out perfectly steamed, and they are ready in just a few minutes.

1 cup water

4 large portobello mushroom caps, brushed clean

2 teaspoons liquid smoke

2 teaspoons maple syrup

½ teaspoon sea salt

4 hamburger buns

4 tomato slices

4 large lettuce leaves

4 onion slices

¼ cup ketchup

¼ cup yellow mustard

1. Pour the water into the pressure cooker pot and insert the trivet.

2. Brush the top of each mushroom cap with ½ teaspoon liquid smoke and ½ teaspoon maple syrup and season with sea salt. Place the mushroom caps on the trivet, stacking if need be.

3. Secure the lid and cook on high pressure for 0 minutes, then quick release the pressure and remove the lid. Press cancel.

4. Set each mushroom cap on a hamburger bun and top with tomato, lettuce, onion, ketchup, and mustard. Serve.

SWITCH IT UP: You can get creative with the toppings for these mushroom burgers; just think of your favorite hamburger toppings.

6 Poultry and Seafood

Shredded Greek Chicken

SERVES 6 TO 8

PREP TIME: 5 MINUTES • COOK TIME: 15 MINUTES • TOTAL TIME: 30 MINUTES

PRESSURE RELEASE: QUICK

ESSENTIAL RECIPE, GLUTEN-FREE, UNDER AN HOUR

Shredded Greek Chicken is a staple in my house. I usually make this one-step "dump and cook" recipe on Sunday night, then store the chicken in the refrigerator to use for various lunches and dinners throughout the week. My family enjoys chicken sliders, Greek salad, lettuce wraps, and Greek pasta. I also use this chicken for chicken gyros, which is my favorite go-to recipe for parties.

2 pounds boneless, skinless chicken breasts

1 cup plain Greek yogurt

½ cup diced red onion

3 tablespoons freshly squeezed lemon juice

3 tablespoons red wine vinegar

2 tablespoons olive oil

2 tablespoons Greek seasoning

2 tablespoons dried dill

1 or 2 garlic cloves, minced

1 teaspoon dried oregano

1. In the inner pot, combine the chicken, yogurt, onion, lemon juice, vinegar, olive oil, Greek seasoning, dried dill, garlic, and oregano.

2. Secure the lid and cook on high pressure for 15 minutes, then quick release the pressure and remove the lid. Press cancel.

3. Remove the chicken from the pot, place it in a medium bowl, and shred it using two forks. Return the chicken to the juices and serve warm.

STORAGE: Refrigerate in a sealed container for up to 3 days or freeze for up to 3 months.

Shredded Smoky Barbecue Chicken

SERVES 6 TO 8

PREP TIME: 5 MINUTES • COOK TIME: 15 MINUTES • TOTAL TIME: 30 MINUTES

PRESSURE RELEASE: QUICK

DAIRY-FREE, UNDER AN HOUR, GLUTEN-FREE

Versatile and perfect for meal-prepping, this tangy barbecue chicken comes together in under an hour. You can use it to make tacos, sandwiches, barbecue chicken pizza, and an array of different salads.

2 pounds boneless, skinless chicken breasts

1 small red onion, diced

1 cup Sweet and Smoky Barbecue Sauce (page 225) or store-bought

2 tablespoons olive oil

1. In the inner pot, combine the chicken, onion, barbecue sauce, and oil.

2. Secure the lid and cook on high pressure for 15 minutes, then quick release the pressure and remove the lid. Press cancel.

3. Remove the chicken from the pot, place it in a medium bowl, and shred it using two forks. Return the chicken to the juices and serve warm.

STORAGE: Refrigerate in a sealed container for up to 3 days or freeze for up to 3 months.

RECIPE TOOLBOX: If you don't have fresh chicken, it's no problem. Frozen chicken can also be used to make this recipe without thawing. Just add 5 minutes to the pressure-cooking time.

Shredded Chinese Five-Spice Chicken Breast

SERVES 6 TO 8
PREP TIME: 5 MINUTES • COOK TIME: 15 MINUTES • TOTAL TIME: 30 MINUTES
PRESSURE RELEASE: QUICK
DAIRY-FREE, GLUTEN-FREE, UNDER AN HOUR

Chinese five-spice adds a spicy-sweet flavor to food, and a little goes a long way. You can use this chicken to make excellent lettuce wraps or a killer stir-fry, and it tastes great over rice or salad. I love making this juicy chicken in my pressure cooker and creating fabulous meals from it all week long.

2 pounds boneless, skinless chicken breasts

1 small red onion, diced

2 tablespoons sesame oil

1 tablespoon Chinese five-spice powder

1. In the inner pot, combine the chicken, onion, sesame oil, and Chinese five-spice.

2. Secure the lid and cook on high pressure for 15 minutes, then quick release the pressure and remove the lid. Press cancel.

3. Remove the chicken from the pot, place it in a medium bowl, and shred it using two forks. Return the chicken to the juices and serve warm.

STORAGE: Refrigerate in a sealed container for up to 3 days or freeze for up to 3 months.

COOK IT SLOW: This recipe can also be easily made in a slow cooker. Simply combine all the ingredients in the slow cooker and cook on low for 6 hours or high for 4 hours. When the chicken is done cooking, shred it with a fork, return it to the juices, and serve or store.

Lemon Chicken Thighs with Capers

SERVES 4
PREP TIME: 12 MINUTES • COOK TIME: 19 MINUTES • TOTAL TIME: 30 MINUTES
PRESSURE RELEASE: QUICK
GLUTEN-FREE, UNDER AN HOUR

Everyone at our dinner table loves the bright taste of lemon, the tangy capers, and chicken cooked to perfection. This dish is the ultimate comfort food, and the cooking process couldn't be simpler: All you need is a few pantry ingredients and 30 minutes to make this crowd-pleasing chicken.

1 tablespoon butter

1 tablespoon olive oil

4 garlic cloves, minced

1 tablespoon capers

1 teaspoon Italian seasoning

6 boneless, skinless chicken thighs

½ cup water

½ cup white wine or water

⅓ cup freshly squeezed lemon juice

1 to 2 teaspoons cornstarch

1. Select sauté and let the pot heat up for 2 minutes.

2. Add the butter, olive oil, garlic, capers, Italian seasoning, and chicken thighs. Sear the chicken thighs for about 2 minutes, or until they are browned on each side. Press cancel. Add the water, wine, and lemon juice to the pot.

3. Secure the lid and cook on high pressure for 12 minutes, then quick release the pressure and remove the lid. Press cancel.

4. Transfer the chicken thighs to a serving dish.

5. Select sauté. Whisk the cornstarch into the pot and whisk for 5 minutes to thicken the sauce.

6. Drizzle the sauce over the chicken thighs and serve.

STORAGE: Refrigerate in an airtight container for up to 5 days or freeze up to 6 months.

MENU PLANNING TIP: These chicken thighs taste lovely when served with Three-Cheese Risotto (page 102) or Parmesan Polenta (page 71).

Maple-Soy Chicken Thighs

SERVES 4

PREP TIME: 12 MINUTES • COOK TIME: 19 MINUTES • TOTAL TIME: 30 MINUTES

PRESSURE RELEASE: QUICK

DAIRY-FREE, UNDER AN HOUR

If you're looking for dinner ideas that please the whole family, try these Maple-Soy Chicken Thighs. My kids always enjoy a dinner that is both savory and sweet, and this dish fits the bill. I love the taste of the sticky maple syrup combined with the ginger's slight spiciness and the salty soy sauce—a mouth-watering combination that makes this dish shine.

¼ cup maple syrup

2 tablespoons soy sauce

2 garlic cloves, minced

1 teaspoon sesame oil

1 teaspoon ground ginger

6 boneless, skinless chicken thighs

1 cup water

1 to 2 teaspoons cornstarch

1. Select sauté. Add the maple syrup, soy sauce, garlic, sesame oil, ginger, and chicken thighs. Cook for 2 minutes, or until the chicken thighs are lightly browned on both sides. Add the water.

2. Secure the lid and cook on high pressure for 12 minutes, then quick release the pressure and remove the lid. Press cancel.

3. Transfer the chicken thighs to a serving dish.

4. Select sauté. Whisk the cornstarch into the pot and whisk for about 5 minutes to thicken the sauce.

5. Drizzle the sauce on top of the chicken thighs and serve.

STORAGE: Refrigerate in an airtight container for up to 5 days or freeze up to 6 months.

MENU PLANNING TIP: These chicken thighs taste great with Sticky Rice (page 68).

Chicken Fajitas

SERVES 4 TO 6
PREP TIME: 10 MINUTES • COOK TIME: 10 MINUTES • TOTAL TIME: 30 MINUTES
PRESSURE RELEASE: QUICK
ONE-POT MEAL, UNDER AN HOUR

These fajitas deliver a "fresh off the grill flavor," all while being a hands-off creation that takes just 30 minutes to cook from start to finish. Enjoy them with guacamole, shredded Cheddar cheese, or sour cream.

For the fajitas

1½ pounds boneless, skinless chicken breasts, cut into long thin strips

1 medium onion, chopped

¾ cup canned crushed tomatoes

¼ cup freshly squeezed lime juice

2 tablespoons vegetable oil

2 teaspoons ground cumin

1 teaspoon chili powder

1 teaspoon smoked paprika

½ teaspoon dried oregano

½ teaspoon cayenne pepper (optional)

3 bell peppers, any color, sliced

For serving

Flour tortillas

Sour cream

Guacamole

Cheddar cheese

To make the fajitas

1. In the inner pot, combine the chicken, onion, tomatoes, lime juice, oil, cumin, chili powder, smoked paprika, oregano, and cayenne (if using).

2. Place a vegetable steamer on top of the chicken and add the bell peppers to the steamer.

3. Secure the lid and cook on high pressure for 7 minutes, then quick release the pressure and remove the lid. Press cancel.

4. Remove the bell peppers and set aside.

5. Select sauté and cook the chicken and onion mixture for about 3 minutes to thicken. Add the bell peppers and toss them in the seasonings.

To serve

6. Set out the tortillas, chicken fajita mixture, sour cream, guacamole, and Cheddar for people to assemble their own fajitas.

COOK IT SLOW: These Chicken Fajitas can easily be adapted to a slow cooker. Place all the ingredients except the bell peppers into a slow cooker. Cook on low for 4 to 6 hours. Add the bell peppers for the last hour.

Creamy Chicken with Cornmeal Dumplings

SERVES 4 TO 6
PREP TIME: 10 MINUTES • COOK TIME: 22 MINUTES • TOTAL TIME: 35 MINUTES
▶ **PRESSURE RELEASE:** NATURAL
ONE-POT MEAL, UNDER AN HOUR

Creamy Chicken with Cornmeal Dumplings will satisfy everyone at your table, especially on a cold day. Tender chicken chunks, savory vegetables, and perfect, slightly sweet cornmeal dumplings couldn't be easier to prepare. After cooking this recipe multiple times, I started placing the dumplings on the trivet on top of the chicken, so the dish doesn't burn. Without the trivet, the dumplings find their way to the bottom of the pan.

For the cornmeal dumplings

1 cup all-purpose flour

1 cup cornmeal

2 tablespoons sugar

½ teaspoon baking powder

½ teaspoon baking soda

½ teaspoon sea salt

½ cup whole milk

1 tablespoon melted butter or olive oil

For the creamy chicken

1 tablespoon butter or olive oil

½ onion, finely chopped

½ cup chopped celery

2 garlic cloves, minced

1 tablespoon herbes de Provence

1½ pounds boneless, skinless chicken breasts, cut into 1-inch chunks

1 (12-ounce) bag frozen mixed vegetables (no need to thaw)

To make the cornmeal dumplings

1. In a large bowl, mix the flour, cornmeal, sugar, baking powder, baking soda, and salt until blended.

2. Add the milk and melted butter, stir until a thick batter forms, and set aside.

To make the creamy chicken

3. Select sauté and let the pot heat up for 2 minutes.

4. Add the butter, onion, celery, garlic, and herbes de Provence. Sauté for 2 minutes, or until the onions are translucent. Press cancel.

5. Add the chicken, frozen vegetables, carrots, chicken stock, and milk.

6. Place a trivet on top of the chicken. Spoon 2-inch dumplings on top of the trivet (you should get 10 to 12).

7. Secure the lid and cook on high pressure for 15 minutes, then allow the pressure to naturally release. Press cancel. Remove the lid and lift out the trivet.

2 carrots, cut into
1-inch chunks

3 cups chicken stock,
store-bought or homemade
(page 223)

1 cup whole milk

1 tablespoon cornstarch

8. Select sauté. Whisk the cornstarch into the pot and whisk for about 5 minutes to thicken the sauce.

9. Add the dumplings to the sauce and serve.

STORAGE: Refrigerate in an airtight container for up to 5 days.

INGREDIENT TIP: Finely ground cornmeal makes the best dumpling dough.

Chicken, Bacon, and Ranch Casserole

SERVES 4
PREP TIME: 5 MINUTES • COOK TIME: 14 MINUTES • TOTAL TIME: 25 MINUTES
PRESSURE RELEASE: QUICK
GLUTEN-FREE, ONE-POT MEAL, UNDER 30 MINUTES

A never-fail casserole is what you need when you want comfort food for your family that will cook super fast. This casserole is an excellent weeknight dinner and also heats up beautifully for lunch. You can use fresh or frozen chicken breasts in this recipe. There is no need to thaw if you use frozen chicken; just put them in whole, then cut into chunks after they are cooked.

3 bacon slices, chopped

½ onion, chopped

1 pound boneless, skinless chicken breasts, cut into 1-inch chunks

1 (12-ounce) bag mixed frozen vegetables (no need to thaw)

2½ cups chicken stock, store-bought or homemade (page 223)

1 cup raw long-grain white rice

1 (1-ounce) packet ranch dressing and seasoning mix

1 cup shredded Cheddar cheese

1. Select sauté and let the pot heat up for 2 minutes.

2. Add the bacon and onion and sauté for about 2 minutes, or until the bacon is halfway crispy and the onions are translucent.

3. Add the chicken, frozen vegetables, chicken stock, rice, and ranch seasoning.

4. Secure the lid and cook on high pressure for 12 minutes, then quick release the pressure and remove the lid. Press cancel.

5. Stir in the Cheddar cheese while the mixture is still piping hot. Serve as soon as the cheese is melted.

STORAGE: Refrigerate in an airtight container for up to 5 days or freeze for up to 6 months.

INGREDIENT TIP: This recipe will have the best results if you use white rice, but brown is lovely, too. If you use brown rice, increase the cooking time to 20 minutes.

Creamy French Mustard Chicken

SERVES 4
PREP TIME: 5 MINUTES • COOK TIME: 10 MINUTES • TOTAL TIME: 35 MINUTES
PRESSURE RELEASE: NATURAL
GLUTEN-FREE, UNDER AN HOUR

Several years ago, my husband and I took a trip to Dijon, France, and we came home with a lot of mustard. Ever since that trip, Dijon mustard has been a pantry staple in my home; I love the tanginess and often use it as a condiment and in recipes. This creamy chicken is cooked in a mouthwatering, savory mustard sauce, and this fancy meal is easy enough for a busy weekday night.

2 tablespoons butter

3 shallots or 1 small onion, chopped

2 garlic cloves, minced

1 cup chicken stock, store-bought or homemade (page 223)

3 tablespoons Dijon mustard

2 teaspoons herbes de Provence

4 (8-ounce) boneless, skinless chicken breasts

Sea salt

Freshly ground black pepper

½ cup heavy (whipping) cream or whole milk

1. Select sauté and let the pot heat up for 2 minutes.

2. Add the butter, shallots, garlic, chicken stock, mustard, and herbes de Provence and stir to make a sauce. Season the chicken breasts with salt and pepper and add them to the pot.

3. Secure the lid and cook on high pressure for 10 minutes, then allow the pressure to naturally release. Press cancel.

4. Remove the lid, stir in the cream, and serve.

STORAGE: Refrigerate in an airtight container for up to 5 days.

MENU PLANNING TIP: This chicken tastes terrific when paired with Cheesy Broccoli (page 61) or Wild Rice with Apples and Shallots (page 70).

Tropical Salsa Chicken Breasts

SERVES 4

PREP TIME: 5 MINUTES • COOK TIME: 10 MINUTES • TOTAL TIME: 25 MINUTES

PRESSURE RELEASE: QUICK

DAIRY-FREE, GLUTEN-FREE, UNDER 30 MINUTES

Pineapple and mango add a refreshing brightness to this dish. Parents will love it because it is made with homemade salsa, and kids will dig it because it incorporates colorful tropical fruit. This fresh and filling recipe is cooked in just minutes, with little prep time, and is a vibrant, nutritious meal. You can serve this chicken over rice for a delicious tropical burrito bowl.

2 pounds boneless, skinless chicken breasts

1 cup Garden Salsa (page 231)

1 cup frozen pineapple chunks (no need to thaw)

1 cup frozen mango chunks (no need to thaw)

½ cup water

1 tablespoon chopped fresh cilantro, for garnish

1. In the inner pot, combine the chicken, salsa, pineapple, mango, and water.

2. Secure the lid and cook on high pressure for 10 minutes, then quick release the pressure and remove the lid. Press cancel.

3. Transfer the chicken to a serving platter. Spoon the salsa and fruit on top of each piece of chicken and garnish with cilantro.

STORAGE: Refrigerate in an airtight container for up to 5 days.

INGREDIENT TIP: Fresh fruit or canned fruit will also work great in this recipe. If you use canned fruit, use the juice from the can in place of the water.

Chicken Caesar Sandwiches

SERVES 4 TO 6
PREP TIME: 5 MINUTES • COOK TIME: 15 MINUTES • TOTAL TIME: 30 MINUTES
PRESSURE RELEASE: QUICK
ONE-POT MEAL, UNDER AN HOUR

I like to whip up these Chicken Caesar Sandwiches for potlucks and anytime my kids have friends over. They only require a few ingredients and make great leftovers. You can make your own Caesar dressing, or you can take a shortcut and use a generous 2 cups of bottled dressing.

For the Caesar dressing

2 cups mayonnaise

4 garlic cloves, minced

¼ cup freshly squeezed lemon juice

2 teaspoons Dijon mustard

2 teaspoons Worcestershire sauce

½ teaspoon sea salt

½ teaspoon freshly ground black pepper

1 teaspoon anchovy paste (optional)

For the chicken

1½ pounds boneless, skinless chicken breasts

1 cup water

1 cup grated Parmesan cheese

For the sandwiches

4 to 6 white sandwich buns

Tomato slices, for serving

Lettuce leaves, for serving

To make the Caesar dressing

1. In a large bowl, combine the mayonnaise, garlic, lemon juice, mustard, Worcestershire sauce, sea salt, pepper, and anchovy paste (if using).

To make the chicken

2. In the inner pot, combine the chicken breasts, Caesar salad dressing, and water.

3. Secure the lid and cook on high pressure for 15 minutes, then quick release the pressure and remove the lid. Press cancel.

4. Remove the chicken, place it in a bowl, and shred it using two forks. Return the chicken to the pot. Stir in the Parmesan.

To make the sandwiches

5. Pile the chicken on the buns and top with tomato and lettuce. Serve.

INGREDIENT TIP: If you use store-bought Caesar salad dressing, stick with creamy Caesar salad dressing to get the right texture.

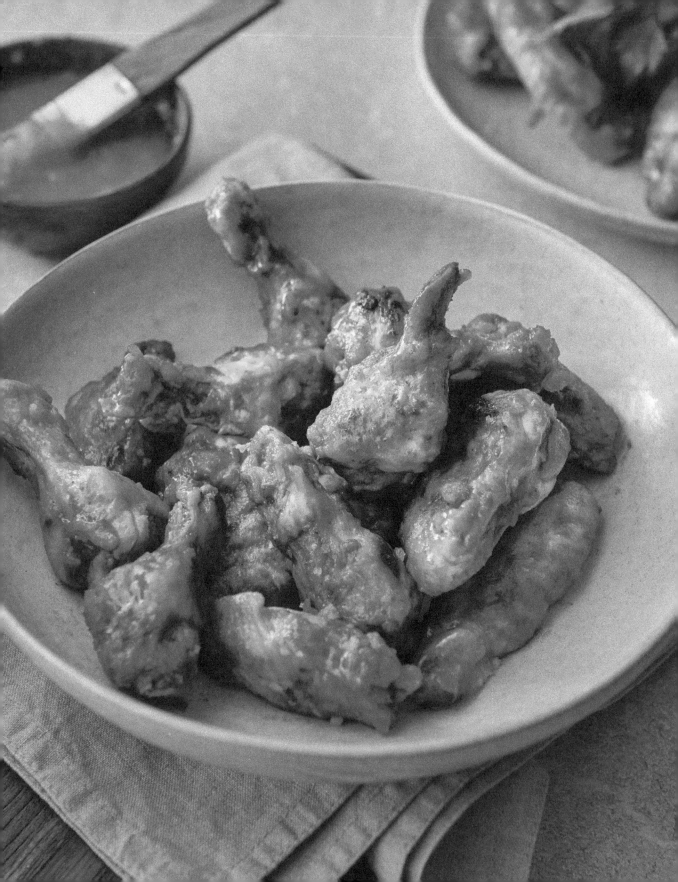

Smoky Barbecue Sticky Chicken Wings

SERVES 4 TO 6

PREP TIME: 5 MINUTES • COOK TIME: 15 MINUTES • TOTAL TIME: 25 MINUTES

PRESSURE RELEASE: QUICK

DAIRY-FREE, GLUTEN-FREE, UNDER 30 MINUTES

On autumn afternoons, I often make an appetizer spread for my family to enjoy while watching college football. Although I need to bring extra napkins when I prepare this recipe, the taste far outweighs the mess. These wings take less time than the premade wings you can purchase from your grocery store's freezer section.

1 cup water

1 cup Sweet and Smoky Barbecue Sauce (page 225)

¼ cup honey

1 small onion, chopped

1 garlic clove, minced

1 teaspoon Worcestershire sauce

2 pounds chicken drumettes or whole wings (tips cut off)

1 tablespoon cornstarch

1. In the inner pot, combine the water, barbecue sauce, honey, onion, garlic, and Worcestershire sauce and whisk together.

2. Place the chicken in a steamer basket. The wings can be stacked, going around the perimeter of the steamer. Add the steamer basket to the pot.

3. Secure the lid and cook on high pressure for 10 minutes, then quick release the pressure and remove the lid. Press cancel.

4. Remove the basket of wings.

5. Select sauté. Whisk the cornstarch into the pot and whisk for about 5 minutes to thicken the sauce.

6. Return the wings to the pot and toss to coat with the sticky barbecue sauce. Serve.

STORAGE: Refrigerate in an airtight container for up to 5 days or freeze for up to 6 months.

SERVING TIP: If you want your wings crispy, place them on a baking sheet and broil them for 5 minutes.

Peanut-Lime Turkey Rice Bowls

SERVES 4

PREP TIME: 15 MINUTES • COOK TIME: 20 MINUTES • TOTAL TIME: 40 MINUTES

PRESSURE RELEASE: QUICK

DAIRY-FREE, ONE-POT MEAL, UNDER AN HOUR

These rice bowls are loaded with creamy, nutty, and gingery flavors, and the lime juice is the perfect finishing touch. You can eat this dish for dinner or lunch, and it also makes for a great appetizer spooned into lettuce leaves. And the best part: You cook the turkey and the rice all in the same pot. (But if you don't want to make rice bowls, you can cook just the ground turkey. See the tip below.)

For the turkey

1½ cups water

½ cup peanut butter

½ onion, chopped

2 garlic cloves, minced

2 tablespoons soy sauce

1 tablespoon sesame oil

1 teaspoon curry powder

1 teaspoon ground ginger

1 pound ground turkey

3 carrots, cut into chunks

1 (8-ounce) can sliced water chestnuts

For the rice

1½ cups water

1 cup raw long-grain white rice

For the bowls

Peanuts

Cilantro

Freshly squeezed lime juice

Sriracha

To make the turkey

1. Select sauté. Add the water, peanut butter, onion, garlic, soy sauce, sesame oil, curry powder, and ground ginger. Stir until well combined.

2. Add the ground turkey, carrots, and water chestnuts and cook the turkey for 5 minutes, breaking it up.

To prepare the rice

3. Add a trivet to the pot.

4. In a 7- to 7½-inch stainless steel bowl, mix the water and rice and place the bowl on the trivet.

5. Secure the lid and cook on high pressure for 12 minutes, then quick release the pressure and remove the lid. Press cancel.

6. Remove the bowl of rice and the trivet.

7. Select sauté. Cook, stirring, for about 3 minutes to thicken the turkey mixture.

To make the bowls

8. Scoop the rice into bowls.

9. Top with the turkey mixture and garnish with peanuts, cilantro, lime juice, and sriracha. Serve.

SWITCH IT UP: You can skip the rice and make just the turkey. Omit the trivet, bowl, rice (and water for the rice). All of the other directions remain the same.

Chimichurri Chicken Drumsticks

SERVES 4
PREP TIME: 5 MINUTES • COOK TIME: 15 MINUTES • TOTAL TIME: 35 MINUTES
PRESSURE RELEASE: QUICK
GLUTEN-FREE, UNDER AN HOUR

These zesty, garlicky, chimichurri drumsticks are so much fun to make and eat. Your taste buds will perk up when you take your first bite of them. Chicken drumsticks are always a hit with my kids and are great to serve when watching the game, or to enjoy on a weeknight. You can take a shortcut and buy your own chimichurri.

8 chicken drumsticks (about 2 pounds total)

1 cup water

½ cup chimichurri, store-bought or homemade (see page 90)

1. In the inner pot, combine the chicken, water, and chimichurri.

2. Secure the lid and cook on high pressure for 15 minutes, then quick release the pressure and remove the lid. Press cancel.

3. Remove the drumsticks and place them on a serving platter. Drizzle the sauce over the chicken and serve.

STORAGE: Refrigerate in an airtight container for up to 5 days or freeze for up to 6 months.

MENU PLANNING TIP: These chicken drumsticks taste wonderful when served with Cauliflower-Potato Mash (page 58).

Spicy Apricot Chicken

SERVES 4

PREP TIME: 5 MINUTES • COOK TIME: 13 MINUTES • TOTAL TIME: 25 MINUTES

PRESSURE RELEASE: QUICK

DAIRY-FREE, UNDER 30 MINUTES

With a sauce that balances sweetness and mild heat, this apricot creation is similar to orange chicken and is a delicious way to get your fix without calling for takeout. You can add more spice if you want, or add less spice if you're serving this chicken to kids. I recommend pairing this recipe with a side of Sticky Rice (page 68).

2 pounds boneless, skinless chicken thighs, cut into strips

1 cup water

¾ cup apricot preserves

2 tablespoons sesame oil

2 tablespoons soy sauce

2 tablespoons rice vinegar

2 teaspoons ground ginger

1 to 2 teaspoons sriracha

1 teaspoon red pepper flakes

2 teaspoons cornstarch

1. In the inner pot, combine the chicken, water, apricot preserves, sesame oil, soy sauce, rice vinegar, ground ginger, sriracha, and red pepper flakes.

2. Secure the lid and cook on high pressure for 8 minutes, then quick release the pressure and remove the lid. Press cancel.

3. Select sauté. Whisk the cornstarch into the pot and whisk for about 5 minutes, until the sauce thickens and becomes sticky.

4. Serve hot.

STORAGE: Refrigerate in an airtight container for up to 5 days.

Turkey Meat Loaf and Mashed Potatoes

SERVES 4 TO 6
PREP TIME: 10 MINUTES • COOK TIME: 25 MINUTES • TOTAL TIME: 50 MINUTES
PRESSURE RELEASE: NATURAL
ONE-POT MEAL, UNDER AN HOUR

When I learned to make meat loaf and mashed potatoes in my electric pressure cooker, whole new culinary worlds opened up. Over the years, I have played around with different meat loaf and glaze recipes. I am going to share my winning meat loaf combination in this dish. Cooking meat loaf in an electric pressure cooker produces moist meat loaf packed with flavor.

For the meat loaf

1 pound ground turkey

1 cup Italian seasoned bread crumbs

½ cup grated Parmesan cheese

1 small onion, finely chopped

1 large egg

2 tablespoons whole milk

For the glaze

½ cup ketchup

1 tablespoon light brown sugar

2 tablespoons Worcestershire sauce

For the mashed potatoes

1 cup water

2 pounds Yukon Gold potatoes, peeled and quartered

2 tablespoons butter

Sea salt

To make the meat loaf

1. In a medium bowl, mix together the ground turkey, bread crumbs, Parmesan, onion, egg, and milk.

To make the glaze

2. In a medium bowl, mix the ketchup, brown sugar, and Worcestershire sauce until blended.

To make the mashed potatoes

3. Pour the water into the pressure cooker pot. Place the potatoes in the water and set a trivet on top of the potatoes.

4. Shape the meat mixture into a loaf (no longer than the width of the trivet) and center it on a 12-inch sheet of heavy-duty aluminum foil. Scrunch up the foil to form a wall around the meat loaf, creating a makeshift loaf pan. (Make sure it will fit in the inner pot.) Spoon the glaze over the meat loaf.

5. Secure the lid and cook on high pressure for 25 minutes, then allow the pressure to naturally release for at least 10 minutes (as the meat loaf will continue cooking during this time). Press cancel.

6. Remove the lid. Lift out the meat loaf and trivet and transfer it to a serving dish.

7. Add the butter and salt to the potatoes, mash them with a fork, and transfer them to a serving bowl.

8. Slice the meat loaf and serve hot with the mashed potatoes.

STORAGE: Refrigerate in an airtight container for up to 5 days.

MENU PLANNING TIP: This meal tastes delicious when paired with Simple Corn on the Cob (page 66).

Sun-Dried Tomato and Olive Turkey Breast

SERVES 4
PREP TIME: 5 MINUTES • COOK TIME: 25 MINUTES • TOTAL TIME: 40 MINUTES
PRESSURE RELEASE: QUICK
DAIRY-FREE, GLUTEN-FREE, UNDER AN HOUR

Serving your family a turkey breast tenderloin is a great way to make dinner-time seem special. My family loves turkey, and the leftovers make fantastic sandwiches for lunch the next day. I added Mediterranean flavors to this recipe to switch things up a bit. Tangy olives, savory sun-dried tomatoes, and sweet basil make this turkey a treat to eat.

1½ pounds turkey breast tenderloin

½ teaspoon sea salt

½ teaspoon freshly ground black pepper

1 cup water

¼ cup dry-pack sun-dried tomatoes, sliced

¼ cup chopped kalamata olives

2 tablespoons dried basil

1 tablespoon olive oil

1. Season the turkey with the salt and pepper.

2. In the inner pot, combine the turkey, water, sun-dried tomatoes, olives, basil, and oil.

3. Secure the lid and cook on high pressure for 25 minutes, then quick release the pressure and remove the lid. Press cancel.

4. Remove the turkey breast and cut it into slices. (If you would like to marinate the flavors into the meat further, select sauté, return the sliced turkey to the sauce, and heat briefly.)

5. Serve the turkey with the juices spooned over it.

STORAGE: Refrigerate in an airtight container for up to 5 days.

MENU PLANNING TIP: Cheesy Broccoli (page 61) is an excellent side dish to serve with this meal.

Turkey Breast with Shallot Gravy

SERVES 4 TO 6
PREP TIME: 15 MINUTES • COOK TIME: 30 MINUTES • TOTAL TIME: 1 HOUR
PRESSURE RELEASE: NATURAL
GLUTEN-FREE

If you're planning a smaller holiday meal, get a small turkey breast and let your electric pressure cooker do the rest of the work for you. This recipe will work for boneless or bone-in turkey breast under 7 pounds. Your family will love the easy gravy made from sweet shallots, and it is so easy, you might find yourself making it all the time.

1 (1½-pound) boneless or bone-in turkey breast

½ teaspoon sea salt

½ teaspoon freshly ground black pepper

2 tablespoons butter

8 shallots, chopped

1 garlic clove, minced

1 teaspoon dried thyme

2 cups water

3 tablespoons cornstarch

1. Season the turkey breast with the salt and pepper.

2. Select sauté and add the butter, shallots, garlic, and thyme. Stir just to melt the butter.

3. Set a trivet in the pot and add the water. Place the turkey breast on the trivet.

4. Secure the lid and cook on high pressure for 25 minutes, then let the pressure naturally release for at least 10 minutes (as the turkey will continue cooking during this time). Press cancel.

5. Remove the lid. Transfer the turkey to a serving dish and remove the trivet from the pot.

6. Select sauté. Whisk the cornstarch into the pot and whisk for about 5 minutes to thicken the gravy.

7. Slice the turkey. Serve the slices drizzled with gravy or pass the gravy separately in a gravy boat.

STORAGE: Refrigerate in an airtight container for up to 5 days.

INGREDIENT TIP: This recipe will work with frozen turkey breast; just add 5 minutes to the cooking time.

Turkey Bolognese

SERVES 4

PREP TIME: 10 MINUTES • COOK TIME: 11 MINUTES • TOTAL TIME: 25 MINUTES

PRESSURE RELEASE: QUICK

DAIRY-FREE, GLUTEN-FREE, UNDER 30 MINUTES

One of the benefits of using an electric pressure cooker is that it produces food that tastes like it has been cooking for hours in a fraction of the time. Bolognese is one of the first things I ever learned how to cook. This hearty sweet and savory Turkey Bolognese tastes like it has been simmering all day long, but the sauce only takes 5 minutes. Try it over angel hair pasta or Parmesan Polenta (page 71).

3 tablespoons olive oil

1 small onion, chopped

3 garlic cloves, minced

1 teaspoon dried basil

1 pound ground turkey

1 (28-ounce) can crushed tomatoes

3 carrots, chopped

1 cup water

½ cup dry red wine

1. Select sauté and let the pot heat up for 2 minutes.

2. Add the olive oil, onion, garlic, and basil and sauté for about 2 minutes, or until the onion is translucent.

3. Add the turkey, tomatoes, carrots, water, and red wine.

4. Secure the lid and cook on high pressure for 5 minutes, then quick release the pressure and remove the lid. Press cancel.

5. Select sauté and cook for an additional 3 to 4 minutes to thicken the sauce, stirring constantly.

STORAGE: Refrigerate in an airtight container for up to 5 days or freeze up to 6 months.

COOK IT SLOW: This sauce can be easily adapted to cook in a slow cooker. Add all the ingredients to a slow cooker and cook for 4 to 6 hours.

Chili-Lime Fish Tacos

SERVES 4
PREP TIME: 5 MINUTES • COOK TIME: 5 MINUTES • TOTAL TIME: 20 MINUTES
PRESSURE RELEASE: QUICK
ONE-POT MEAL, UNDER 30 MINUTES

Every year, during Lent, we make these fish tacos at least once. The chili powder and lime juice combination will make your taste buds celebrate. The fish requires just a few ingredients and steams in your electric pressure cooker in a few short minutes. You can use any white fish for this recipe. I like serving these tacos in warmed, soft corn tortillas with crunchy cabbage.

For the fish

1 cup water

1 tablespoon smoked paprika

1 tablespoon chili powder

1 teaspoon sea salt

1½ pounds fresh cod fillets

3 tablespoons freshly squeezed lime juice

1 teaspoon vegetable oil

For the tacos

8 corn tortillas, warmed

1 (16-ounce) bag coleslaw mix

1 cup Garden Salsa (page 231)

1 avocado, chopped

½ cup shredded Cotija cheese

To make the fish

1. Pour the water into the inner pot and insert the trivet.

2. In a medium bowl, mix the smoked paprika, chili powder, and salt. Rub the spice mixture on the cod and drizzle the fish with the lime juice and oil.

3. Arrange the pieces of fish on the trivet.

4. Secure the lid and cook on high pressure for 5 minutes, then quick release the pressure and remove the lid. Press cancel.

To make the tacos

5. Remove the fish and divide into 8 portions. Top the warmed tortillas with fish and garnish with the coleslaw, salsa, avocado, and Cotija. Serve.

INGREDIENT TIP: You can make this recipe using frozen fish if you add 2 minutes to the cooking time. No thawing is necessary.

Mussels in Marinara Sauce

SERVES 4

PREP TIME: 5 MINUTES • COOK TIME: 3 MINUTES • TOTAL TIME: 20 MINUTES

PRESSURE RELEASE: QUICK

DAIRY-FREE, GLUTEN-FREE, UNDER 30 MINUTES

You might think you are in a nice Italian restaurant when these fragrant mussels are placed on the table. Who knew mussels could be made at home in mere minutes? This variety of shellfish can be intimidating for a home cook, but I am here to tell you that this is one of the easiest meals one can make in an electric pressure cooker.

2 tablespoons olive oil

1 onion, chopped

2 garlic cloves, minced

2 pounds mussels, scrubbed and debearded

2½ cups Marinara Sauce (page 232)

½ cup water

1 tablespoon Italian seasoning

1. Select sauté and let the pot heat up for 2 minutes.

2. Add the olive oil, onion, and garlic and sauté for about 2 minutes, or until the onion is translucent. Press cancel.

3. Add the mussels, marinara sauce, water, and Italian seasoning.

4. Secure the lid and cook on high pressure for 1 minute, then quick release the pressure and remove the lid.

5. Transfer the mussels and the sauce to a bowl and serve.

MENU PLANNING TIP: These mussels are delicious when served with spaghetti.

Steamed Honey-Garlic Salmon

SERVES 4

PREP TIME: 5 MINUTES • COOK TIME: 8 MINUTES • TOTAL TIME: 25 MINUTES

PRESSURE RELEASE: QUICK

GLUTEN-FREE, UNDER 30 MINUTES

Salmon steamed in the electric pressure cooker might be my kids' favorite meal, especially this honey-garlic creation. They get so excited when they find out this salmon is for supper, and it has become a dinner staple in our home. This salmon turns out sweet, garlicky, and bright. I have added instructions for frozen salmon as well as fresh; no thawing is necessary.

4 (5-ounce) skinless salmon fillets

Sea salt

Freshly ground black pepper

2 tablespoons olive oil

2 tablespoons freshly squeezed lemon juice

2 tablespoons honey

3 garlic cloves, minced

1 cup water

1. Season the salmon fillets with salt and pepper. Place the fish on a flat surface and top each fillet with olive oil, lemon juice, honey, and garlic.

2. Pour the water into the inner pot and insert a trivet. Arrange the salmon on the trivet.

3. Secure the lid and cook on high pressure for 8 minutes (add about 5 minutes for fillets that are more than 1½ inches thick), then quick release the pressure and remove the lid. Press cancel.

4. Remove the salmon from the trivet and serve.

MENU PLANNING TIP: This salmon tastes excellent with Salted Baby Potatoes (page 60).

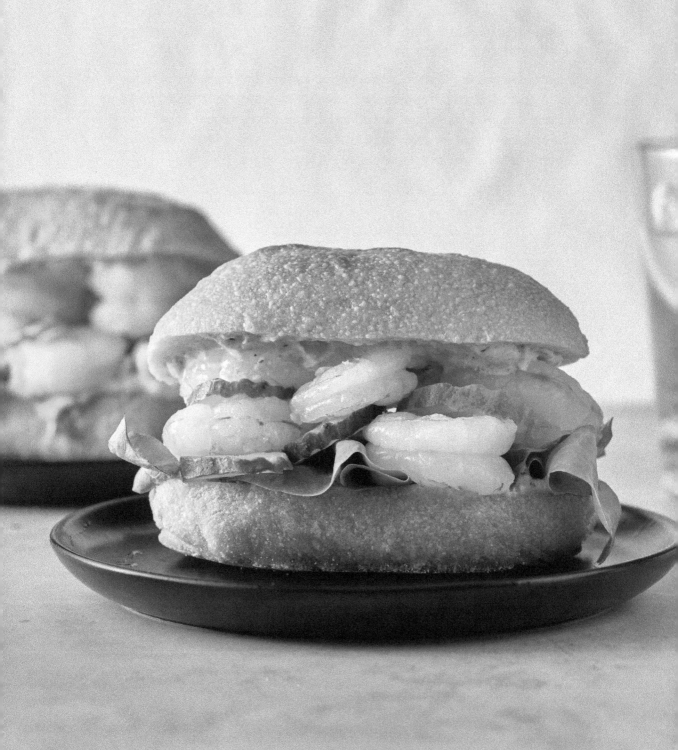

Po' Boy Shrimp Sandwiches

SERVES 4
PREP TIME: 5 MINUTES • COOK TIME: 1 MINUTE • TOTAL TIME: 15 MINUTES
PRESSURE RELEASE: QUICK
DAIRY-FREE, ONE-POT MEAL, UNDER 30 MINUTES

Po' Boy Shrimp Sandwiches are made of a few delicious ingredients but are packed with a smoky, spicy flavor that will wow your taste buds. Once in a while, my husband and I enjoy making these sandwiches for an "at-home date night" while we send the kids downstairs to watch a movie. These electric pressure cooker sandwiches couldn't be easier to make, and you don't even need to thaw the shrimp.

For the rémoulade sauce

¼ cup mayonnaise

¼ cup horseradish sauce

½ teaspoon garlic powder

½ teaspoon smoked paprika

½ teaspoon Cajun seasoning

For the sandwiches

12 ounces peeled and deveined shrimp, fresh or frozen

1 tablespoon freshly squeezed lemon juice

1 tablespoon Cajun seasoning

1 cup water

4 white sandwich buns

2 dill pickles, sliced

4 large lettuce leaves

To make the rémoulade sauce

1. In a small bowl, mix the mayonnaise, horseradish sauce, garlic powder, smoked paprika, and Cajun seasoning until well blended.

2. Set the sauce aside.

To make the sandwiches

3. In a medium bowl, toss the shrimp with the lemon juice and Cajun seasoning.

4. Add the water to the inner pot. Place the seasoned shrimp in a steamer basket and place the basket in the pot.

5. Secure the lid and cook on high pressure for 0 minutes if using fresh shrimp or 1 minute if using frozen shrimp. Quick release the pressure and remove the lid.

6. Spread 2 tablespoons of rémoulade sauce on each bun. Add the shrimp, pickles, and lettuce and serve.

INGREDIENT TIP: I recommend McCormick Cajun seasoning.

Steamed Orange-Ginger Halibut

SERVES 4

PREP TIME: 5 MINUTES • COOK TIME: 8 MINUTES • TOTAL TIME: 25 MINUTES

PRESSURE RELEASE: QUICK

DAIRY-FREE, GLUTEN-FREE, UNDER 30 MINUTES

This halibut is an extremely low-maintenance recipe that calls for only four ingredients (not counting salt and pepper). It will turn out flaky and sweet, and the ground ginger adds a little spice. My kids love a little sweetness with fish, and they're always enthusiastic about eating this dish.

¼ cup orange marmalade

2 teaspoons ground ginger

4 (5-ounce) halibut fillets

2 teaspoons vegetable oil

Sea salt

Freshly ground black pepper

1 cup water

1. In a small bowl, mix together the orange marmalade and ground ginger.

2. Brush each piece of halibut with vegetable oil and season with salt and pepper.

3. Place the orange marmalade-ginger mixture on top of each piece of halibut.

4. Pour the water into the inner pot and insert the trivet. Taking care not to let the marmalade slide off (using tongs helps), arrange the fish on the trivet.

5. Secure the lid and cook on high pressure for 8 minutes, then quick release the pressure and remove the lid. Press cancel.

6. Remove the fish from the trivet using tongs and serve.

INGREDIENT TIP: You can make this recipe using frozen halibut if you add 2 extra minutes to the cooking time.

Mediterranean Tuna Noodle Casserole

SERVES 4
PREP TIME: 5 MINUTES • COOK TIME: 6 MINUTES • TOTAL TIME: 25 MINUTES
PRESSURE RELEASE: QUICK
ONE-POT MEAL, UNDER 30 MINUTES

Adding Mediterranean flavors to traditional tuna noodle casserole is a great way to give this classic Midwestern dish a face-lift. My kids love any meal with the name casserole in it. This is creamy, comforting, rich-tasting, and incredibly easy to prepare. Grab a few Mediterranean staples out of your pantry and throw this lovely dish together pronto.

2 cups water

2 cups whole milk

12 ounces rotini

2 (4.5-ounce) cans oil-packed tuna, undrained

1 small onion, chopped

2 garlic cloves, minced

¼ cup chopped marinated artichoke hearts

2 tablespoons chopped sun-dried tomatoes, dry-pack or oil-packed

1 teaspoon Italian seasoning

1 tablespoon capers

1 cup shredded mozzarella cheese

½ cup grated Parmesan cheese

1. In the inner pot, combine the water, milk, rotini, tuna (with the oil from the cans), onion, garlic, artichoke hearts, sun-dried tomatoes, Italian seasoning, and capers. Push the pasta down to be sure it is completely submerged in the liquid.

2. Secure the lid and cook on high pressure for 6 minutes, then quick release the pressure and remove the lid. Press cancel.

3. While the noodles are still piping hot, stir in the mozzarella and Parmesan cheeses. Serve as soon as the cheese is completely melted.

STORAGE: Refrigerate in an airtight container for up to 5 days.

INGREDIENT TIP: Both dried sun-dried tomatoes or oil-packed work in this recipe.

7 Pork, Beef, and Lamb

Basic Cola Pulled Pork

SERVES 6

PREP TIME: 5 MINUTES • COOK TIME: 45 MINUTES • TOTAL TIME: 1 HOUR 10 MINUTES

▶ **PRESSURE RELEASE:** NATURAL

DAIRY-FREE, ESSENTIAL RECIPE, GLUTEN-FREE, WORTH THE WAIT

My family adores this simple pulled pork recipe because it makes delicious sandwiches. Pork was actually one of the first things I learned how to make in my electric pressure cooker, and this version tastes better than pork that has been simmering in a slow cooker all day. Use this smoky, pleasantly sweet pork as the star ingredient in barbecue pizza, lettuce wraps, salad, or sandwiches.

2 pounds boneless pork loin roast

Sea salt

Freshly ground black pepper

1 cup Sweet and Smoky Barbecue Sauce (page 225)

1 (12-ounce) can cola

1 onion, chopped

2 garlic cloves, minced

2 tablespoons Worcestershire sauce

1. Season the pork with salt and pepper.

2. In the inner pot, combine the pork, barbecue sauce, cola, onion, garlic, and Worcestershire sauce.

3. Secure the lid and cook on high pressure for 45 minutes, then allow the pressure to naturally release for at least 10 minutes (as the pork will continue cooking during this time). Press cancel.

4. Remove the lid, transfer the pork to a medium bowl, and shred it using two forks. Return the pork to the juices and serve.

STORAGE: Refrigerate in a sealed container for up to 5 days or freeze for up to 6 months.

COOK IT SLOW: This recipe and the following pulled pork dishes can be adapted for a slow cooker. Simply add all the ingredients to a slow cooker. Cook on low for 8 hours and shred the pork at the end.

Basic Salsa Pulled Pork

SERVES 6
PREP TIME: 5 MINUTES • COOK TIME: 45 MINUTES • TOTAL TIME: 1 HOUR
10 MINUTES
PRESSURE RELEASE: NATURAL
DAIRY-FREE, GLUTEN-FREE, WORTH THE WAIT

Salsa pulled pork is an excellent meal to serve at parties. I get compliments on this recipe every time I make it, and people hardly believe it when I tell them it is only four ingredients. This pulled pork also works wonderfully for meal prep because you can make it ahead and freeze when you need a fast meal. Try it with delicious tacos, enchiladas, quesadillas, lettuce wraps, and salads.

1 tablespoon vegetable oil

2 pounds boneless pork loin roast

3½ cups Garden Salsa (page 231)

1 (1-ounce) packet taco seasoning

1. In the inner pot, combine the vegetable oil, pork, salsa, and taco seasoning.

2. Secure the lid and cook on high pressure for 45 minutes, then allow the pressure to naturally release for at least 10 minutes (as the pork will continue cooking during this time). Press cancel.

3. Remove the lid, transfer the pork to a medium bowl, and shred it using two forks. Return the pork to the juices and serve.

STORAGE: Refrigerate in a sealed container for up to 5 days or freeze for up to 6 months.

INGREDIENT TIP: You can also use store-bought salsa in this recipe. My favorite brand is Frontera fire-roasted tomato salsa.

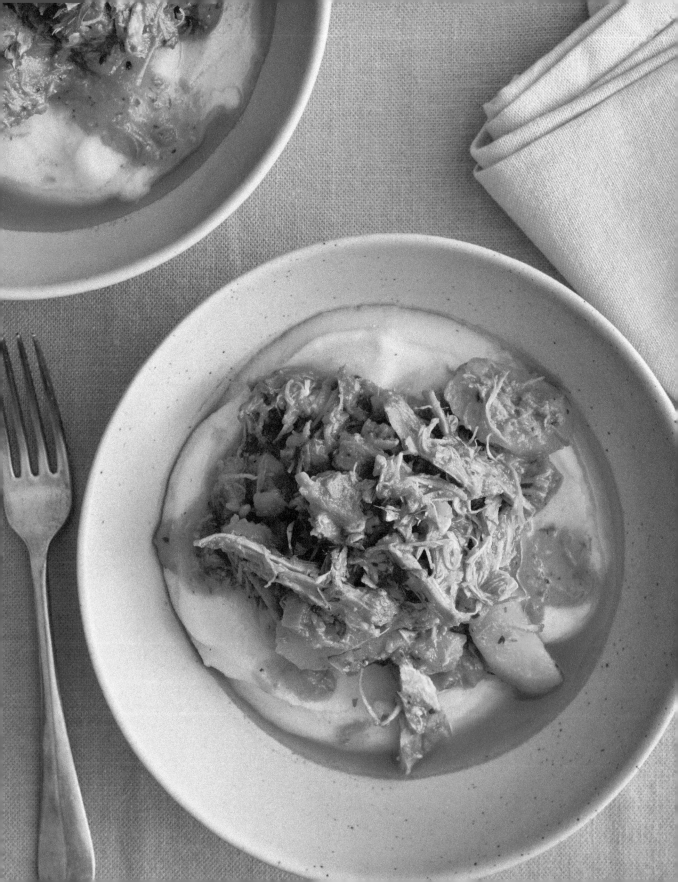

Pulled Pork Ragu

SERVES 6
PREP TIME: 5 MINUTES • COOK TIME: 45 MINUTES • TOTAL TIME: 1 HOUR
10 MINUTES
PRESSURE RELEASE: NATURAL
DAIRY-FREE, GLUTEN-FREE, WORTH THE WAIT

In my house, we love Italian food. Once in a while, I find us in a "jarred marinara sauce" rut, and this ragu is the perfect solution to our dilemma. This pork ragu is savory, sweet, and has a short ingredient list. I love serving this sauce over noodles or polenta, and it makes great leftovers, too.

1 tablespoon olive oil

1½ pounds pork tenderloin, cut into 3-inch chunks

1 (28-ounce) can crushed tomatoes

½ cup water

3 carrots, cut into ½-inch chunks

3 shallots or 1 small onion, chopped

3 garlic cloves, minced

1 tablespoon Italian seasoning

1. In the inner pot, combine the olive oil, pork, crushed tomatoes, water, carrots, shallots, garlic, and Italian seasoning.

2. Secure the lid and cook on high pressure for 45 minutes, then allow the pressure to naturally release for at least 10 minutes (as the pork will continue cooking during this time). Press cancel.

3. Remove the lid, transfer the pork to a medium bowl, and shred it using two forks. Return the pork to the juices and serve.

STORAGE: Refrigerate in a sealed container for up to 5 days or freeze for up to 6 months.

MENU PLANNING TIP: This ragu tastes awesome on Parmesan Polenta (page 71).

Basic Apple Cider Pulled Pork

SERVES 6

PREP TIME: 5 MINUTES • COOK TIME: 45 MINUTES • TOTAL TIME: 1 HOUR
10 MINUTES

PRESSURE RELEASE: NATURAL

DAIRY-FREE, GLUTEN-FREE, WORTH THE WAIT

When I start to see apple cider hit the shelves in the fall, I always pick up
a container so that I can make this dish. Apple cider pulled pork is a really
delicious way to switch up the basic recipe. Try it on slider buns for a perfect
autumn meal to enjoy while watching football. If apple cider is out of season,
you can also use hard apple cider in this recipe.

2 pounds boneless pork
loin roast

Sea salt

Freshly ground black pepper

1 tablespoon vegetable oil

2 cups apple cider

2 Honeycrisp apples, peeled
and sliced

1 small onion, chopped

1 tablespoon light
brown sugar

1 teaspoon chili powder

1 teaspoon smoked paprika

1. Season the pork with salt and pepper.

2. In the inner pot, combine the vegetable oil, pork,
apple cider, apples, onion, brown sugar, chili
powder, and smoked paprika.

3. Secure the lid and cook on high pressure for
45 minutes, then allow the pressure to naturally
release for at least 10 minutes (as the pork will
continue cooking during this time). Press cancel.

4. Remove the lid, transfer the pork to a medium
bowl, and shred it using two forks. Return the
pork to the juices and serve.

STORAGE: Refrigerate in a sealed container for
up to 5 days or freeze for up to 6 months.

COOK IT SLOW: This recipe can be adapted for
a slow cooker. Simply add all the ingredients to a
slow cooker and cook on low for 8 hours. Shred the
pork at the end.

Cinnamon Applesauce Pork Chops

SERVES 6
PREP TIME: 10 MINUTES • COOK TIME: 12 MINUTES • TOTAL TIME: 40 MINUTES
PRESSURE RELEASE: NATURAL
DAIRY-FREE, GLUTEN-FREE, UNDER AN HOUR

Tender pork cooked in applesauce is a comforting meal and the definition of fall perfection. This easy dinner is flavorful, tender, and kid-friendly. My kids love applesauce, and this meal makes an appearance on our dinner table a few times every fall season. Even better, since this is a "dump and cook recipe," you can throw it together in a pinch for a weeknight dinner.

6 (6- to 8-ounce) boneless pork chops (1 inch thick)

Sea salt

Freshly ground black pepper

1 tablespoon vegetable oil

1 small onion, chopped

1½ cups applesauce, store-bought or homemade (page 233)

1 cup water

1 teaspoon dried sage

1 cinnamon stick

1. Season the pork chops with salt and pepper.

2. Select sauté and let the pot heat up for 2 minutes.

3. Pour the oil into the pot, then add the onion and sauté for about 2 minutes, or until the onion is translucent. Add the pork chops and sear for 1 minute on each side.

4. Add the applesauce, water, sage, and cinnamon stick.

5. Secure the lid and cook on high pressure for 10 minutes, then let the pressure naturally release. Press cancel.

6. Remove the lid and transfer the pork chops to a serving dish. Discard the cinnamon stick, scoop the applesauce on top of the pork, and serve.

STORAGE: Refrigerate in a sealed container for up to 5 days.

COOK IT SLOW: This recipe can easily be adapted for a slow cooker. Sauté the onions and season and sear the pork on the stovetop, then place them in a slow cooker with the water, applesauce, sage, and cinnamon stick. Cook on low for 4 to 6 hours.

Large-Batch Smoky Barbecue Pork Chop Sandwiches

SERVES 10
PREP TIME: 5 MINUTES • COOK TIME: 22 MINUTES • TOTAL TIME: 45 MINUTES
▶ **PRESSURE RELEASE:** NATURAL
ONE-POT MEAL, UNDER AN HOUR

When I want to welcome a visitor to the Midwest, I bring them to a town festival where they serve pork chop sandwiches. Boneless pork chops cook up fast in the electric pressure cooker, and you can serve dinner to a crowd in under an hour. This recipe is perfect for families because you will have enough leftovers for lunch the next day. They are sweet, smoky, and the definition of Midwestern perfection on a bun.

For the pork

1 tablespoon butter

1 small onion, chopped

2 garlic cloves, minced

10 (8-ounce) boneless pork chops (1 inch thick)

1 cup Sweet and Smoky Barbecue Sauce (page 225) or store-bought

1 cup water

½ cup packed light brown sugar

1 tablespoon Worcestershire sauce

1 tablespoon apple cider vinegar

For the sandwiches

10 hamburger buns

1 head lettuce, separated into large lettuce leaves

3 tomatoes, sliced

½ cup yellow mustard

Sliced pickles

To make the pork

1. Select sauté and let the pot heat up for 2 minutes.

2. Add the butter, onion, and garlic and sauté for 2 minutes, or until the onion is translucent.

3. Add the pork chops, barbecue sauce, water, brown sugar, Worcestershire sauce, and vinegar.

4. Secure the lid and cook on high pressure for 20 minutes, then allow the pressure to naturally release for at least 10 minutes (as the pork will continue cooking during this time). If desired, leave the pressure cooker on the "keep warm" setting and use the pot as a serving vessel.

To make the sandwiches

5. Set out the buns and all the fixings and let people assemble their own sandwiches.

STORAGE: Refrigerate in a sealed container for up to 5 days.

COOK IT SLOW: This recipe will adapt easily to a slow cooker. Sauté the onions and garlic on the stovetop, then place the sautéed onions and garlic in a slow cooker with the rest of the ingredients. Cook on low for 4 to 6 hours.

Herbes de Provence Pork Chops

SERVES 4 TO 6

PREP TIME: 10 MINUTES • COOK TIME: 14 MINUTES • TOTAL TIME: 40 MINUTES

PRESSURE RELEASE: NATURAL

DAIRY-FREE, GLUTEN-FREE, UNDER AN HOUR

Herbes de Provence paired with Dijon mustard, garlic, and lemon juice might be my ultimate favorite flavor profile. The French herb blend contains all the herbs I love—rosemary, thyme, marjoram, basil, and lavender. When you cook up these pork chops, your taste buds will do a happy dance. They are fancy enough to serve for a holiday meal but achievable for any night of the week. This recipe is always a massive hit with my family.

¼ cup freshly squeezed lemon juice

3 tablespoons Dijon mustard

2 tablespoons herbes de Provence

2 tablespoons olive oil

1 small onion, chopped

1 tablespoon minced garlic

4 to 6 (4-ounce) boneless pork chops (½ inch thick)

Sea salt

Freshly ground black pepper

1 cup water

1 tablespoon cornstarch

1. Select sauté. Add the lemon juice, mustard, herbes de Provence, olive oil, onion, and garlic. Whisk for 1 minute, until well blended.

2. Season the pork chops with salt and pepper and add to the pot along with the water.

3. Secure the lid and cook on high pressure for 8 minutes, then allow the pressure to naturally release. Press cancel.

4. Remove the lid and transfer the pork chops to a serving dish.

5. Select sauté. Whisk the cornstarch into the pot and whisk for about 5 minutes to thicken the sauce.

6. Pour the sauce on top of the pork chops and serve.

STORAGE: Refrigerate in a sealed container for up to 5 days.

MENU PLANNING TIP: I enjoy serving these pork chops with Wild Rice with Apples and Shallots (page 70).

Sesame-Ginger Pork Tenderloin

SERVES 4 TO 6
PREP TIME: 10 MINUTES • COOK TIME: 23 MINUTES • TOTAL TIME: 45 MINUTES
PRESSURE RELEASE: NATURAL
DAIRY-FREE, UNDER AN HOUR

This recipe combines all my favorite Chinese-inspired flavors such as ginger, garlic, sweet hoisin sauce, and salty soy sauce. I enjoy serving this pork loin over rice, with lo mein noodles, on a salad, or as an entrée with a few side dishes. Skip the takeout and make this healthy dish at home instead.

½ cup hoisin sauce

2 tablespoons light brown sugar

1 tablespoon sesame oil

1 tablespoon soy sauce

1 tablespoon rice vinegar

2 teaspoons ground ginger

2 garlic cloves, minced

1½ pounds pork tenderloin

Sea salt

Freshly ground black pepper

1 cup water

1 tablespoon cornstarch

1. Select sauté. Add the hoisin sauce, brown sugar, sesame oil, soy sauce, rice vinegar, ground ginger, and garlic. Whisk for about 3 minutes, until a sauce forms.

2. Season the pork tenderloin with salt and pepper. Add the pork tenderloin and water.

3. Secure the lid and cook on high pressure for 15 minutes, then allow the pressure to naturally release for at least 10 minutes (as the pork will continue cooking during this time). Press cancel.

4. Remove the lid and transfer the pork to a cutting board.

5. Select sauté. Whisk the cornstarch into the pot and whisk for about 5 minutes to thicken the sauce.

6. Slice the pork and serve with the sauce poured over it.

STORAGE: Refrigerate in a sealed container for up to 5 days.

MENU PLANNING TIP: I enjoy serving this pork tenderloin with a side of Farro (page 67).

Pork Tenderloin with Pepper Jelly Glaze

SERVES 4 TO 6

PREP TIME: 10 MINUTES • COOK TIME: 20 MINUTES • TOTAL TIME: 45 MINUTES

PRESSURE RELEASE: NATURAL

DAIRY-FREE, GLUTEN-FREE, UNDER AN HOUR

Pepper jelly pork tenderloin turns out flavorful and tender when cooked in an electric pressure cooker. The sweet and spicy pepper jelly produces a delicious glaze that pairs well with the tender white meat. All ages will love the sweet and slightly spicy pork, and it is excellent for leftovers like sliders for lunch the next day.

½ cup apple juice

½ cup hot pepper jelly

2 tablespoons apple cider vinegar

1½ pounds pork tenderloin

Sea salt

Freshly ground black pepper

½ cup water

1½ teaspoons cornstarch

1. In the inner pot, combine the apple juice, hot pepper jelly, and vinegar. Whisk together until a sauce forms.

2. Season the pork with salt and pepper and add the pork tenderloin and water to the pot.

3. Secure the lid and cook on high pressure for 15 minutes, then allow the pressure to naturally release. Press cancel.

4. Remove the lid and transfer the pork to a cutting board.

5. Select sauté. Add the cornstarch and whisk until the sauce thickens, about 5 minutes.

6. Slice the pork and serve with the sauce on top.

STORAGE: Refrigerate in a sealed container for up to 5 days.

INGREDIENT TIP: Tabasco brand pepper jelly works well in this recipe.

Smoky Barbecue Ribs

SERVES 4 TO 6
PREP TIME: 10 MINUTES • COOK TIME: 30 MINUTES • TOTAL TIME: 55 MINUTES
PRESSURE RELEASE: NATURAL
DAIRY-FREE, GLUTEN-FREE, UNDER AN HOUR

There is no need to get out the smoker or the grill if you want to make some delicious barbecue ribs. These electric pressure cooker barbecue ribs are fall-off-the-bone tender and super juicy. Since you can cook spectacular ribs so easily, enjoy a delectable rack any night of the week during any time of the year.

2 tablespoons light brown sugar

2 tablespoons smoked paprika

1 teaspoon cayenne pepper (optional)

1 (4-pound) rack pork back ribs, shiny membrane removed

1 cup water

1 cup Sweet and Smoky Barbecue Sauce (page 225) or store-bought

1 onion, chopped

3 garlic cloves, minced

1 tablespoon Worcestershire sauce

1. In a small bowl, mix together the brown sugar, smoked paprika, and cayenne (if using) and rub the spice mixture all over the ribs.

2. In the inner pot, combine the water, barbecue sauce, onion, garlic, and Worcestershire sauce. Fold the ribs into the pot. You can also cut them up if you like.

3. Secure the lid and cook on high pressure for 25 minutes, then allow the pressure to naturally release. Press cancel.

4. Remove the lid and transfer the ribs to a serving platter.

5. Select sauté and cook the sauce for 5 minutes to thicken. Brush the sauce on the ribs and serve.

STORAGE: Refrigerate in a sealed container for up to 5 days.

SERVING TIP: If you want your ribs crispy, broil them in the oven for about 3 minutes before serving.

Sausage and Peppers

SERVES 4

PREP TIME: 10 MINUTES • COOK TIME: 20 MINUTES • TOTAL TIME: 35 MINUTES

PRESSURE RELEASE: QUICK

DAIRY-FREE, GLUTEN-FREE, UNDER AN HOUR

Sausage and peppers remind me of home. Growing up in Chicagoland, I have had my fair share of sausage and peppers. It was important to me to learn how to make this dish to get my fix now that I live in a different state. I usually serve this Sausage and Peppers on a bun as a sandwich, but they are delicious on their own as well.

1 (28-ounce) can crushed tomatoes

½ cup water

5 links sweet Italian sausage, halved

1 onion, sliced

2 garlic cloves, minced

1 tablespoon Italian seasoning

4 bell peppers, any color, cut into strips

1. In the inner pot, combine the crushed tomatoes, water, sausages, onion, garlic, and Italian seasoning.

2. Place the peppers in a vegetable steamer and add it to the pot on top of the sausage mixture.

3. Secure the lid and cook on high pressure for 15 minutes, then quick release the pressure and remove the lid. Press cancel.

4. Remove the steamer of bell peppers from the pot.

5. Select sauté and cook for about 5 minutes to thicken the sauce.

6. Return the bell peppers to the pot, stir them into the sauce, and serve.

STORAGE: Refrigerate in a sealed container for up to 5 days.

MENU PLANNING TIP: Sausage and peppers taste delicious when served on toasted Italian bread.

Sweet Orange Ham

SERVES 4 TO 6
PREP TIME: 5 MINUTES • COOK TIME: 20 MINUTES • TOTAL TIME: 35 MINUTES
PRESSURE RELEASE: NATURAL
GLUTEN-FREE, UNDER AN HOUR

My family often serves this dish for our holiday gatherings, but after I figured out how easy it was to prepare ham in my electric pressure cooker, I started making ham for lunch sandwiches. A ham cooks to perfection in under 40 minutes, and your family will be impressed when you serve this for dinner on a random Wednesday. I have also included instructions (see tip) for cooking a frozen ham with no thawing needed.

1 cup orange juice

½ cup water

2 tablespoons butter

1 (3- to 4-pound) spiral-cut ham

½ cup packed light brown sugar

1 teaspoon ground cinnamon

1 teaspoon ground cloves

1 teaspoon ground nutmeg

1 tablespoon cornstarch

1. In the inner pot, combine the orange juice, water, and butter.

2. Rub the ham all over with the brown sugar, cinnamon, cloves, and nutmeg.

3. Place the trivet in the pressure cooker pot and set the ham on the trivet.

4. Secure the lid and cook on high pressure for 15 minutes, then allow the pressure to naturally release. Press cancel.

5. Remove the lid and carefully lift out the ham and trivet. Select sauté. Whisk the cornstarch into the pot and whisk for about 5 minutes to thicken the sauce.

6. Serve the ham drizzled with the sauce.

STORAGE: Refrigerate in a sealed container for up to 5 days.

SWITCH IT UP: To cook a frozen ham, increase the cooking time to 30 minutes.

Cheesy Chili Mac

SERVES 4 TO 6

PREP TIME: 10 MINUTES • COOK TIME: 10 MINUTES • TOTAL TIME: 25 MINUTES

PRESSURE RELEASE: QUICK

ONE-POT MEAL, UNDER 30 MINUTES

This dish might be the most frequent round-two recipe I prepare in my house. We make chili a lot during the winter months, and what's not to love about a comforting recipe that is fabulous repurposed into a delicious pasta? This chili mac is saucy, sweet, and cheesy and is super simple to throw together. The following recipe makes chili from scratch, but if you have leftover chili, see the tip below for how to use it here.

For the chili

1 pound ground beef

1 small onion, chopped

1 (15-ounce) can kidney beans, drained and rinsed

1 (15-ounce) can tomato sauce

1 tablespoon chili powder

1 teaspoon ground cumin

For the mac

3 cups water

12 ounces elbow macaroni

1 tablespoon butter

3 cups shredded Cheddar cheese

½ cup whole milk

To make the chili

1. Select sauté and let the pot heat up for 2 minutes.

2. Add the ground beef and onions and cook for about 5 minutes to brown the meat and soften the onions. Press cancel and stir the meat and onions so that nothing is sticking to the bottom of the pot. Add the kidney beans, tomato sauce, chili powder, and cumin.

To make the mac

3. Add the water, macaroni, and butter to the chili in the pot, making sure the macaroni is submerged in the liquid.

4. Secure the lid and cook on high pressure for 5 minutes, then quick release the pressure and remove the lid. Press cancel.

5. Add the Cheddar cheese while the noodles are still piping hot.

6. Stir in the milk and serve.

STORAGE: Refrigerate in a sealed container for up to 5 days.

RECIPE TOOLBOX: If you have 4 cups of leftover chili, you can skip the made-from-scratch chili here. Omit the chili ingredients and steps 1 and 2. When making the mac, add the 4 cups of leftover chili to the pot along with the water, macaroni, and butter. Proceed with the recipe as written.

Sloppy Joes

SERVES 4 TO 6
PREP TIME: 10 MINUTES • COOK TIME: 12 MINUTES • TOTAL TIME: 35 MINUTES
PRESSURE RELEASE: NATURAL
DAIRY-FREE, ONE-POT MEAL, UNDER AN HOUR

I shied away from making sloppy joes in my electric pressure cooker at first because they don't take long when you do them on the stove. I am so happy I tried them because they taste like they have been slow cooking all day. I promise you will love them. Sloppy joes are a staple in my house, and they are an incredibly comforting meal any time of the year. This recipe makes great leftovers, but I doubt that you will have any.

1 pound ground beef

1 small onion, chopped

½ cup chopped celery

1 (8-ounce) can tomato sauce

¼ cup ketchup

2 tablespoons light brown sugar

2 teaspoons Worcestershire sauce

1 teaspoon garlic powder

6 hamburger buns

1. Select sauté and let the pot heat up for 2 minutes.

2. Add the ground beef, onion, and celery. Brown the beef for about 3 minutes, but don't worry about cooking it all the way. Press cancel.

3. Add the tomato sauce, ketchup, brown sugar, Worcestershire sauce, and garlic powder.

4. Secure the lid and cook on high pressure for 5 minutes, then allow the pressure to naturally release. Press cancel and remove the lid.

5. Select sauté and cook for 2 to 4 minutes to thicken the sauce.

6. Scoop the sloppy joes onto the buns and serve.

STORAGE: Refrigerate in a sealed container for up to 5 days.

MENU PLANNING TIP: Cheesy Broccoli (page 61) would make an excellent side dish.

Beef and Broccoli

SERVES 4 TO 6

PREP TIME: 10 MINUTES • COOK TIME: 13 MINUTES • TOTAL TIME: 40 MINUTES
PRESSURE RELEASE: NATURAL
DAIRY-FREE, UNDER AN HOUR

Your entire family will ask for this tasty Beef and Broccoli. It is healthier than takeout and tastes better, too, especially over Sticky Rice (page 68). This homemade version will impress everyone, and you will have one happy family when you present this meal on a busy night.

¾ cup fresh tangerine juice

¼ cup soy sauce

3 tablespoons light brown sugar

2 tablespoons sesame oil

3 garlic cloves, minced

1 teaspoon ground ginger

1 pound stewing beef, cut into ½-inch-wide strips

1 tablespoon cornstarch

1 (12-ounce) bag microwaveable broccoli florets

1. In the inner pot, combine the tangerine juice, soy sauce, brown sugar, sesame oil, garlic, and ginger. Whisk the ingredients together until well combined.

2. Add the beef to the pot.

3. Secure the lid and cook on high pressure for 8 minutes, then allow the pressure to naturally release. Press cancel and remove the lid.

4. Select sauté. Whisk the cornstarch into the pot and whisk for about 5 minutes to thicken the sauce.

5. Steam the broccoli in the microwave and add it to the beef and sauce. Serve.

STORAGE: Refrigerate in a sealed container for up to 5 days.

SWITCH IT UP: You can make this recipe gluten-free by substituting tamari sauce for the soy sauce.

Sesame Beef with Sugar Snap Peas

SERVES 4 TO 6
PREP TIME: 10 MINUTES • COOK TIME: 16 MINUTES • TOTAL TIME: 40 MINUTES
PRESSURE RELEASE: NATURAL
DAIRY-FREE, UNDER AN HOUR

In this recipe, the electric pressure cooker turns an inexpensive cut—stew meat—into wonderfully tender beef accented by a slightly sweet ginger-laced sauce. You can use a high-grade beef cut if you like, but there's really no need to. I add the sugar snap peas right at the end, so they stay crunchy.

¾ cup water

¼ cup soy sauce

3 garlic cloves, minced

3 tablespoons light brown sugar

2 tablespoons sesame oil

1 teaspoon ground ginger

1 pound stewing beef, cut into ½-inch-wide strips

1 tablespoon cornstarch

8 ounces sugar snap peas

¼ cup chopped scallions, green part only

1 tablespoon sesame seeds

1. In the inner pot, combine the water, soy sauce, garlic, brown sugar, sesame oil, and ginger. Whisk the ingredients together until well combined. Add the meat.

2. Secure the lid and cook on high pressure for 8 minutes, then allow the pressure to naturally release. Press cancel and remove the lid.

3. Select sauté. Whisk the cornstarch into the pot and whisk for about 5 minutes to thicken the sauce.

4. Add the sugar snap peas and toss with the meat for about 3 minutes with the heat still on. Press cancel.

5. Serve topped with the scallion greens and sesame seeds.

MENU PLANNING TIP: This dish is excellent over Sticky Rice (page 68), Brown Rice (page 72), or Farro (page 67).

Thai Beef and Potato Curry

SERVES 4 TO 6
PREP TIME: 10 MINUTES • COOK TIME: 8 MINUTES • TOTAL TIME: 40 MINUTES
PRESSURE RELEASE: NATURAL
DAIRY-FREE, GLUTEN-FREE, UNDER AN HOUR

I tried making this Thai Beef and Potato Curry for years, and it took me a while before I got it right. I have learned that using full-fat coconut milk in Thai curry recipes is a must. I also like to sweeten mine up by adding pineapple. This is a dreamy and colorful meal to serve when you want something a little different. I have tried cooking this recipe on my stovetop several times, but it turns out so much better in the electric pressure cooker.

1 tablespoon vegetable oil

1 pound stewing beef, cut into 1-inch chunks

3 or 4 Yukon Gold potatoes, cut into 2-inch chunks

2 (15-ounce) cans full-fat coconut milk

¼ cup Thai red curry paste

2 tablespoons sugar

1 teaspoon ground turmeric

1 cup frozen pineapple chunks, thawed

Sticky Rice (page 68), for serving

¼ cup chopped scallions

¼ cup chopped peanuts

1. In the inner pot, combine the vegetable oil, meat, potatoes, coconut milk, curry paste, sugar, and turmeric.

2. Secure the lid and cook on high pressure for 8 minutes, then allow the pressure to naturally release. Press cancel.

3. Remove the lid and stir in the pineapple.

4. Serve over the rice, topped with the scallions and chopped peanuts.

STORAGE: Refrigerate in a sealed container for up to 5 days.

INGREDIENT TIP: I recommend the Thai Kitchen brand coconut milk.

Steak Gyros

SERVES 4 TO 6
PREP TIME: 10 MINUTES • COOK TIME: 10 MINUTES • TOTAL TIME: 40 MINUTES
PRESSURE RELEASE: NATURAL
ONE-POT MEAL, UNDER AN HOUR

If you're looking for something to serve for a special occasion, I highly recommend Steak Gyros. I love serving gyros when hosting a get-together in my home. There is nothing quite like perfectly seasoned tender steak served on warm pita bread and topped with vegetables and creamy tzatziki sauce.

For the tzatziki sauce

1 cup plain yogurt, store-bought or homemade (page 228)

1 small English cucumber, chopped

2 garlic cloves, minced

2 teaspoons dried or fresh dill

½ teaspoon freshly squeezed lemon juice

Dash sea salt

For the steak

1 tablespoon olive oil

1 pound skirt or flank steak, cut into ½-inch-wide strips

1 red onion, chopped

½ cup beef stock, store-bought or homemade (page 224)

4 garlic cloves, minced

1 teaspoon dried marjoram

1 teaspoon dried oregano

1 teaspoon Greek seasoning

To make the tzatziki sauce

1. In a medium bowl, mix the yogurt, cucumber, garlic, dill, lemon juice, and salt until well combined. Cover and marinate in the refrigerator for 30 minutes.

To cook the steak

2. Select sauté and let the pot heat up for 2 minutes.

3. Add the oil, steak, and onions and cook for about 2 minutes, or until the onion is translucent.

4. Add the beef stock, garlic, marjoram, oregano, and Greek seasoning.

5. Secure the lid and cook on high pressure for 8 minutes, then allow the pressure to naturally release. Press cancel.

6. Remove the lid and transfer the meat to a bowl.

For the gyros

4 to 6 pita breads or naan, warmed

1 red onion, chopped

1 tomato, sliced

½ cup crumbled feta cheese

½ cup sliced kalamata olives

To make the gyros

7. Spoon the tzatziki sauce into a warmed pita bread. Top with the steak, onion, tomato slices, feta, and olives and serve.

STORAGE: Refrigerate in a sealed container for up to 5 days or freeze for up to 6 months.

MENU PLANNING TIP: This steak can also be served over a salad. The tzatziki sauce makes a delicious salad dressing!

French Onion Pot Roast

SERVES 4 TO 6
PREP TIME: 10 MINUTES • COOK TIME: 42 MINUTES • TOTAL TIME: 1 HOUR
20 MINUTES
PRESSURE RELEASE: QUICK
DAIRY-FREE, ONE-POT MEAL, WORTH THE WAIT

Pot roast is a dish that involves minimal prep time and just a few ingredients but builds enormous flavor. Although this French onion version takes a little over an hour to make, that time is relatively fast compared to most slow cooker versions. This is a delicious classic that is ideal for Sunday night supper. I have included potatoes and carrots here, but if you want to make just the roast, pressure-cook it for 40 minutes (20 minutes per pound).

1 tablespoon olive oil

3 onions, sliced

2 pounds beef roast, such as rump or chuck

Sea salt

Freshly ground black pepper

1 cup water

¼ cup soy sauce

2 tablespoons Worcestershire sauce

1 teaspoon Dijon mustard

1 pound Yukon Gold potatoes, peeled and quartered

4 carrots, cut into 2-inch chunks

1. Select sauté and let the pot heat up for 2 minutes.

2. Add the olive oil and onions and cook for about 2 minutes, or until the onions are translucent.

3. Season the roast with salt and pepper. Add it to the pot and sear on all sides.

4. Add the water, soy sauce, Worcestershire sauce, and mustard.

5. Secure the lid and cook on high pressure for 30 minutes, then quick release the pressure and remove the lid. Press cancel.

6. Set a collapsible vegetable steamer over the roast. Place the potatoes and carrots on the steamer.

7. Secure the lid and cook on high pressure for 10 minutes, then quick release the pressure and remove the lid. Check to make sure that the internal temperature of the beef is 160°F.

8. Slice the roast and serve with the pot juices and onions drizzled over, with the vegetables on the side. (Keep any sliced meat in the remaining onions and juices to keep it moist.)

STORAGE: Refrigerate in a sealed container for up to 5 days.

COOK IT SLOW: This recipe can be adapted to a slow cooker. Simply cook the onions and sear the beef roast on the stovetop, place the roast, onions, and other ingredients into the slow cooker (including the potatoes and carrots), and cook on high for 6 hours or on low for 8 hours.

Short Ribs with Butter and Muffuletta

SERVES 4 TO 6
PREP TIME: 10 MINUTES • COOK TIME: 37 MINUTES • TOTAL TIME: 55 MINUTES
PRESSURE RELEASE: NATURAL
GLUTEN-FREE, UNDER AN HOUR

Once in a while, my husband and I like to have an at-home date night. We cook something fancy and eat a quiet meal together without the kids. These delectable short ribs always fit the bill. The olive salad traditionally used to make muffuletta sandwiches is my favorite condiment: It is a perfect mixture of Italian pickled vegetables and olives tossed in olive oil, and it pairs incredibly with beef. Cooking short ribs in an electric pressure cooker is super easy, and they turn out fantastic.

4 pounds beef short ribs

Sea salt

Freshly ground black pepper

2 tablespoons butter

1 small onion, chopped

2 garlic cloves, minced

1 cup water

½ cup muffuletta (Italian olive salad)

1. Select sauté and let the pot heat up for 2 minutes.

2. Season the ribs with salt and pepper.

3. Add the butter, onion, and garlic to the pot and cook for about 2 minutes, or until the onions are translucent. Add the ribs and sear them on each side, about 5 minutes in total.

4. Add the water and muffuletta.

5. Secure the lid and cook on high pressure for 30 minutes, then allow the pressure to naturally release. Press cancel.

6. Remove the lid and transfer the ribs to a serving dish. Top them with the muffuletta sauce and serve.

STORAGE: Refrigerate in a sealed container for up to 5 days.

INGREDIENT TIP: I recommend the olive muffuletta from That Pickle Guy (spelled "muffalata" on their label).

Chimichurri Beef Tips

SERVES 4 TO 6
PREP TIME: 5 MINUTES • COOK TIME: 12 MINUTES • TOTAL TIME: 35 MINUTES
PRESSURE RELEASE: NATURAL
DAIRY-FREE, GLUTEN-FREE, UNDER AN HOUR

Beef tips cook up in tangy, zesty chimichurri in no time and produce big flavor. You can make this recipe with stewing meat or a higher-grade cut like top sirloin steak or flank steak. I love serving these beef tips over rice, in a sandwich wrap, or over a salad.

1 tablespoon olive oil

1½ pounds stewing beef, cut into ½-inch-wide strips

½ onion, chopped

½ cup water

½ cup chimichurri, store-bought or homemade (see page 90)

1. Select sauté and let the pot heat up for 2 minutes.

2. Add the oil, beef, and onion and sauté for about 2 minutes to brown the beef and soften the onion. There is no need to cook the meat all the way through.

3. Add the water and chimichurri.

4. Secure the lid and cook on high pressure for 10 minutes, then allow the pressure to naturally release. Press cancel.

5. Remove the lid and transfer the beef and sauce to a serving dish and serve.

STORAGE: Refrigerate in a sealed container for up to 5 days.

Roast Beef Sundaes with Horseradish

SERVES 4 TO 6

PREP TIME: 10 MINUTES • **COOK TIME:** 35 MINUTES • **TOTAL TIME:** 50 MINUTES

PRESSURE RELEASE: QUICK

GLUTEN-FREE, ONE-POT MEAL, UNDER AN HOUR

This unusual recipe is a Midwest classic and the ultimate comfort food. A roast beef sundae looks similar to an ice cream sundae, but it is made with all savory food items. My kids love this meal, and we never have leftovers. This recipe is an easy one-pot meal that will please the entire family and is a snap to prepare for a weeknight.

For the beef

1 tablespoon vegetable oil

2 pounds beef rump roast, cut into 3-inch chunks

1 onion, chopped

2 garlic cloves, minced

2 cups beef stock, store-bought or homemade (page 224), or water

⅓ cup horseradish sauce

1 bay leaf

For the mashed potatoes

2 pounds Yukon Gold potatoes, peeled and halved

2 tablespoons butter

Sea salt

Freshly ground black pepper

For the sundaes

½ cup shredded Cheddar cheese

½ cup sour cream

¼ cup chopped scallions, green part only

4 to 6 cherry tomatoes

To prepare the beef

1. Select sauté and let the pot heat up for 2 minutes.

2. Add the oil, beef, onions, and garlic and sauté for 5 minutes to brown the meat and soften the onions.

3. Add the beef stock, horseradish sauce, and bay leaf. Press cancel.

To prepare the mashed potatoes

4. Place a vegetable steamer over the beef. You will have to adjust the food so that the steamer fits in the pot. Add the potatoes to the steamer.

5. Secure the lid and cook on high pressure for 30 minutes, then quick release the pressure and remove the lid. Press cancel.

6. Transfer the potatoes to a large bowl, add the butter, smash with a fork, and season with salt and pepper.

7. Discard the bay leaf. Shred the beef directly in the pot and stir it into the juices.

To assemble the sundaes

8. Scoop the mashed potatoes into individual bowls. Top with the beef, Cheddar cheese, sour cream, and scallions. Set a cherry tomato on top and serve.

STORAGE: Refrigerate the meat mixture in a sealed container for up to 5 days.

INGREDIENT TIP: I cut the beef roast into chunks to shorten the cooking time, but also so that the potatoes and the beef can cook together in the same pot.

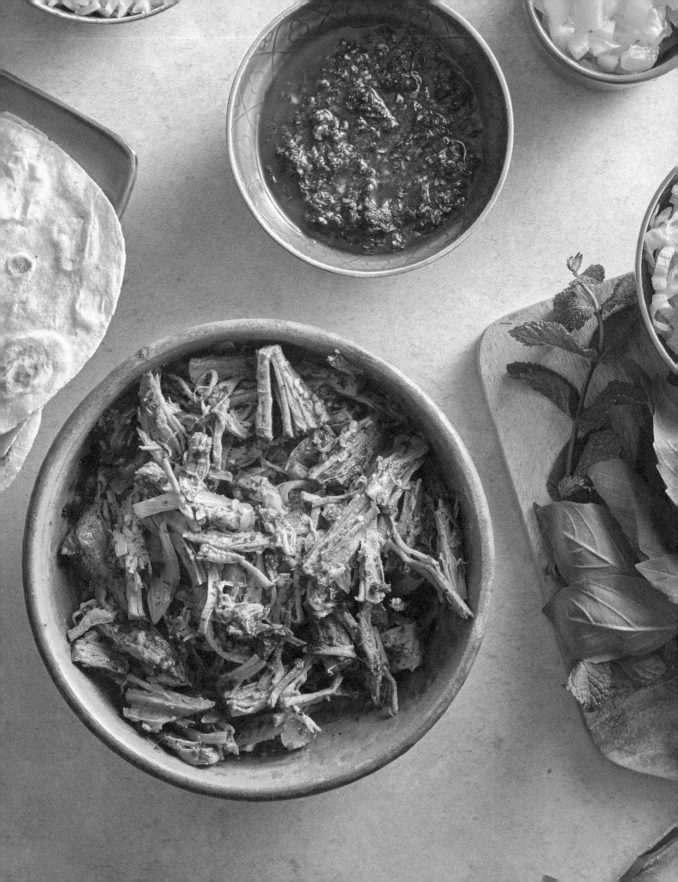

Salsa Verde Beef Tacos

SERVES 6 TO 10
PREP TIME: 10 MINUTES • COOK TIME: 72 MINUTES • TOTAL TIME: 1 HOUR
40 MINUTES
PRESSURE RELEASE: NATURAL
ONE-POT MEAL, WORTH THE WAIT

When I want melt-in-your-mouth tender shredded beef, I cook the beef roast in my electric pressure cooker for a long time. Beef roasts will cook through in a shorter amount of time, but if you want beef that will pull apart at the touch of a fork, it takes at least 70 minutes. This amount of time is still short when compared to cooking a roast in the slow cooker, and the finished product is out of this world. You can add all of your favorite taco toppings if you like, but they're not needed because this beef is so flavorful.

For the beef

1 tablespoon olive oil

5 garlic cloves, minced

1 onion, sliced

3 pounds chuck roast

Sea salt

Freshly ground black pepper

2½ cups salsa verde

1 cup beef stock, store-bought or homemade (page 224) or water

For the tacos

6 to 10 (8-inch) soft flour tortillas

¼ cup shredded Cheddar cheese

½ cup sour cream

1 cup shredded lettuce

1 medium tomato, sliced

To make the beef

1. Select sauté and let the pot heat up for 2 minutes.

2. Add the oil, garlic, and onion and sauté for about 2 minutes, or until the onion is translucent.

3. Season the roast with salt and pepper, add it to the pot, and sear on all sides. Add the salsa and beef stock.

4. Secure the lid and cook on high pressure for 70 minutes, then allow the pressure to naturally release. Press cancel.

5. Remove the lid and use two forks to shred the beef right in the pot. Let the shredded meat marinate in the sauce. If desired, set the cooker to "keep warm" and serve the beef right out of the pot.

CONTINUED

To make the tacos

6. Set out the shredded beef, tortillas, Cheddar cheese, sour cream, lettuce, and tomato and let people build their own tacos.

STORAGE: Refrigerate the beef in a sealed container for up to 5 days.

MENU PLANNING TIP: You can make delicious grain bowls using this shredded beef. I like serving it over Farro (page 67).

Garlic and Rosemary Lamb Chops

SERVES 6
PREP TIME: 10 MINUTES • COOK TIME: 10 MINUTES • TOTAL TIME: 30 MINUTES
PRESSURE RELEASE: NATURAL
DAIRY-FREE, GLUTEN-FREE, UNDER AN HOUR

Lamb chops turn out tender, luscious, and evenly cooked when you make them in the electric pressure cooker. This meal is fancy enough for a special occasion, but easy enough that there's no reason to stress about it. These lamb chops are a restaurant-quality meal you can easily make at home.

2 tablespoons olive oil

3 shallots or 1 small onion, chopped

2 garlic cloves, minced

3 tablespoons freshly squeezed lemon juice

1 teaspoon dried oregano

1 teaspoon Greek seasoning

6 lamb loin chops (2 inches thick)

Sea salt

Freshly ground black pepper

1 cup water

1. Select sauté and let the pot heat up for 2 minutes.

2. Add the olive oil, shallots, garlic, lemon juice, oregano, and Greek seasoning. Season the lamb with salt and pepper, add to the pan, and sear for 1 minute on each side.

3. Add the water. Secure the lid and cook on high pressure for 8 minutes, then allow the pressure to naturally release. Press cancel.

4. Remove the lid and transfer the lamb to serving plates. Spoon the pan juices over the lamb and serve.

> **MENU PLANNING TIP:** These lamb chops taste excellent when served with Green Beans with Shallots and Bacon (page 65).

Ground Lamb Shepherd's Pie

SERVES 4 TO 6
PREP TIME: 10 MINUTES • COOK TIME: 27 MINUTES • TOTAL TIME: 40 MINUTES
PRESSURE RELEASE: QUICK
GLUTEN-FREE, ONE-POT MEAL, UNDER AN HOUR

Shepherd's pie is fabulous comfort food and will warm you up on a cold day. Made from mostly kitchen staples, this is my go-to recipe when I want to make a meal for a new mom or family in need. When I am gifting it, I arrange it in a casserole dish to make it look presentable, but when I make this meal for my family, I just serve it straight out of the pot.

For the filling

1 tablespoon olive oil

1 small onion, chopped

3 garlic cloves, minced

2 teaspoons herbes de Provence

1 pound ground lamb

2 carrots, chopped

1 cup frozen corn kernels (no need to thaw)

1 cup frozen peas (no need to thaw)

2 cups beef stock, store-bought or homemade (page 224)

2 tablespoons tomato paste

2 tablespoons Worcestershire sauce

1 tablespoon cornstarch

For the topping

2 pounds Yukon Gold potatoes, peeled and cut into 2-inch chunks

2 tablespoons butter

Sea salt

Freshly ground black pepper

To make the filling

1. Select sauté and let the pot heat up for 2 minutes.

2. Add the olive oil, onion, garlic, and herbes de Provence and sauté for about 2 minutes, or until the onion is translucent.

3. Add the ground lamb and cook for about 5 minutes, or until browned. You don't have to worry about cooking it all the way.

4. Add the carrots, corn, peas, beef stock, tomato paste, and Worcestershire sauce. Press cancel.

To make the topping

5. Place a vegetable steamer over the lamb and vegetables and place the potatoes in the steamer.

6. Secure the lid and cook on high pressure for 15 minutes, then quick release the pressure and remove the lid. Press cancel.

7. Transfer the potatoes to a large bowl, add the butter, smash with a fork, and season with salt and pepper.

8. Select sauté. Whisk the cornstarch into the meat and vegetables and cook for 5 minutes to thicken the sauce. Press cancel.

9. Spoon the potatoes on top of the lamb and serve.

STORAGE: Refrigerate in a sealed container for up to 5 days.

SWITCH IT UP: You can easily make this recipe with ground beef instead of ground lamb. And if you want a browned topping for the potatoes, spoon the meat mixture into a baking dish, spread the mashed potatoes on top, and run under the broiler to brown.

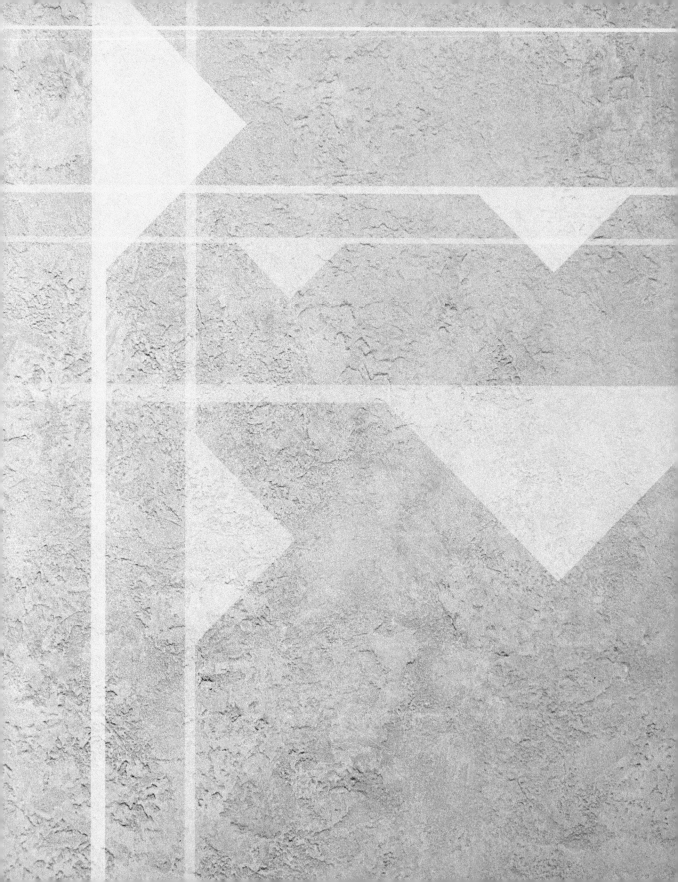

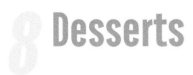

Desserts

Vanilla Cheesecake

SERVES 6 TO 10
PREP TIME: 10 MINUTES • COOK TIME: 35 MINUTES • TOTAL TIME: 1 HOUR
5 MINUTES, PLUS 6 TO 8 HOURS TO CHILL
▶ **PRESSURE RELEASE:** NATURAL
ESSENTIAL RECIPE, VEGETARIAN, WORTH THE WAIT

I never thought that making cheesecake at home was attainable until I dove into the world of electric pressure cookers. Cheesecake turns out silky and smooth, and it cooks perfectly. It is essential to carefully follow the cooking method, but once you get acquainted with this process, you will want to bring cheesecake to every holiday gathering.

For the crust

Nonstick cooking spray

8 full graham cracker sheets, crushed

3 tablespoons butter, melted

For the cheesecake

16 ounces full-fat cream cheese, at room temperature

½ cup sour cream, at room temperature

¾ cup sugar

½ teaspoon sea salt

2 tablespoons pure vanilla extract

1 teaspoon freshly squeezed lemon juice

1 tablespoon cornstarch

3 large eggs

1 cup water

To make the crust

1. Line the bottom of a 7-inch springform pan with a round of parchment paper or mist the pan with cooking spray.

2. In a medium bowl, mix the graham cracker crumbs and melted butter together and press the mixture evenly into the bottom and about ½ inch up the sides of the springform pan.

To make the cheesecake

3. In a medium bowl, with an electric mixer or by hand, beat the cream cheese, sour cream, sugar, salt, vanilla, lemon juice, and cornstarch until well blended. Beat in the eggs just until incorporated. Do not overmix.

4. Spoon the cream cheese mixture into the springform pan and cover the pan with foil.

5. Pour the water into the pot and insert a trivet or a silicone sling (if you don't have a sling or a trivet with handles, fashion a foil sling and place it on the trivet). Place the springform pan on the trivet or sling.

6. Secure the lid and cook on high pressure for 35 minutes, then allow the pressure to naturally release. Press cancel and remove the lid.

7. Carefully lift out the pan using the handles of the trivet or sling. Refrigerate the cheesecake for 6 to 8 hours to chill and set up.

8. Uncover and remove the sides of the pan. Cut the cheesecake into slices and serve.

STORAGE: Refrigerate in a sealed container for up to 3 days.

INGREDIENT TIP: I recommend using Kirkland pure vanilla extract.

Lemon Cheesecake

SERVES 6 TO 10
PREP TIME: 10 MINUTES • COOK TIME: 35 MINUTES • TOTAL TIME: 1 HOUR
5 MINUTES, PLUS 6 TO 8 HOURS TO CHILL
▶ **PRESSURE RELEASE:** NATURAL
VEGETARIAN, WORTH THE WAIT

I try to add citrus to my desserts whenever I have the chance. This Lemon Cheesecake is super refreshing and is the perfect summer dessert. It turns out creamy and bright and has the perfect amount of sweetness. My husband loves cheesecake, so I enjoy making this every year for his summertime birthday.

For the crust

Nonstick cooking spray

8 graham crackers, crushed

3 tablespoons butter, melted

For the cheesecake

16 ounces full-fat cream cheese, at room temperature

½ cup sour cream, at room temperature

¾ cup sugar

½ teaspoon sea salt

1 tablespoon cornstarch

Grated zest of 2 lemons

1 tablespoon freshly squeezed lemon juice

3 large eggs

1 cup water

To make the crust

1. Line the bottom of a 7-inch springform pan with a round of parchment paper or mist the pan with cooking spray.

2. In a medium bowl, mix the graham cracker crumbs and melted butter together and press the mixture evenly into the bottom of the springform pan.

To make the cheesecake

3. In a medium bowl, with a hand mixer or by hand, beat together the cream cheese, sour cream, sugar, salt, cornstarch, lemon zest, and lemon juice.

4. Beat in the eggs just until incorporated. Do not overmix.

5. Spoon the cream cheese mixture into the spring-form pan and cover the pan with foil.

6. Pour the water into the pot and insert a trivet or a silicone sling (if you don't have a sling or a trivet with handles, fashion a foil sling and place it on the trivet). Place the springform pan on the trivet or sling.

7. Secure the lid and cook on high pressure for 35 minutes, then allow the pressure to naturally release. Press cancel and remove the lid.

8. Carefully lift out the pan using the handles of the trivet or sling. Refrigerate the cheesecake for 6 to 8 hours to chill and set up.

9. Uncover and remove the sides of the pan. Cut the cheesecake into slices and serve.

STORAGE: Refrigerate in a sealed container for up to 3 days.

SWITCH IT UP: Make the crust with different cookie crumbs, such as vanilla wafers.

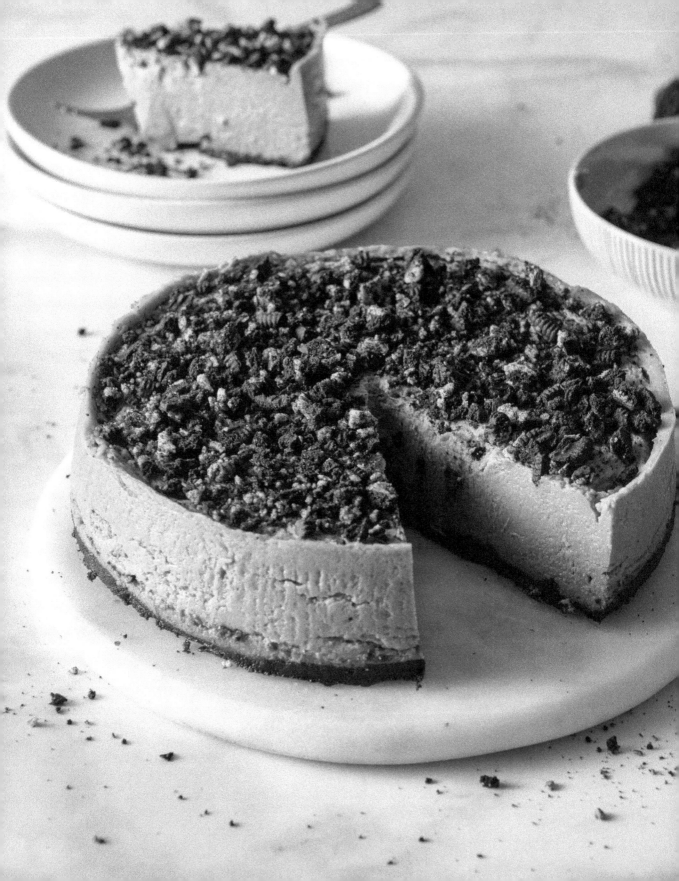

Chocolate Cookie Cheesecake

SERVES 6 TO 10
PREP TIME: 10 MINUTES • COOK TIME: 35 MINUTES • TOTAL TIME: 1 HOUR
5 MINUTES, PLUS 6 TO 8 HOURS TO CHILL
PRESSURE RELEASE: NATURAL
VEGETARIAN, WORTH THE WAIT

This version of cheesecake is smooth, silky, rich, and chocolaty and will impress everyone. It is the perfect dessert to make for your chocolate-loving friends and ideal to bring for any gathering. This recipe tastes so much better than the "no-bake" boxed cheesecake mixes you find in stores.

For the crust

Nonstick cooking spray

½ cup chocolate sandwich cookie crumbs

3 tablespoons butter, melted

For the cheesecake

16 ounces full-fat cream cheese, at room temperature

½ cup sour cream, at room temperature

¾ cup sugar

2 tablespoons unsweetened cocoa powder

½ teaspoon sea salt

2 tablespoons pure vanilla extract

1 tablespoon cornstarch

3 large eggs

1 cup water

½ cup chocolate sandwich cookie crumbs, for topping

To make the crust

1. Line the bottom of a 7-inch springform pan with a round of parchment paper or mist the pan with cooking spray.

2. In a medium bowl, mix the cookie crumbs and melted butter together and press the mixture evenly into the bottom of the springform pan.

To make the cheesecake

3. In a medium bowl, with a hand mixer or by hand, beat the cream cheese, sour cream, sugar, cocoa, salt, vanilla, and cornstarch until well blended.

4. Beat in the eggs just until incorporated. Do not overmix.

5. Spoon the cream cheese mixture into the springform pan and cover the pan with foil.

6. Pour the water into the pot and insert a trivet or a silicone sling (if you don't have a sling or a trivet with handles, fashion a foil sling and place it on the trivet). Place the springform pan on the trivet or sling.

CONTINUED

7. Secure the lid and cook on high pressure for 35 minutes, then allow the pressure to naturally release. Press cancel and remove the lid.

8. Carefully lift out the pan using the handles of the trivet or sling. Refrigerate the cheesecake for 6 to 8 hours to chill and set up.

9. Uncover and remove the sides of the pan. Top with the cookie crumbs, cut into slices, and serve.

STORAGE: Refrigerate in a sealed container for up to 3 days.

INGREDIENT TIP: I recommend Ghirardelli Dutch process cocoa for this recipe.

Cinnamon-Apple Rice Pudding

SERVES 6
PREP TIME: 5 MINUTES • COOK TIME: 15 MINUTES • TOTAL TIME: 30 MINUTES
PRESSURE RELEASE: QUICK
GLUTEN-FREE, UNDER AN HOUR, VEGETARIAN

I have many people in my family who are gluten-free. This rice pudding has graced our Thanksgiving dessert table for the last several years for them. It is incredibly easy to prepare and is so comforting and delicious. If you reduce the sugar in this recipe, you can turn it into a lovely cold-weather breakfast recipe.

2 cups whole milk

1 cup long-grain white rice

1 cup water

1 cup chopped peeled apples

½ cup sugar

1 tablespoon pure vanilla extract

1 cinnamon stick

1 large egg

1 cup half-and-half

1. In the inner pot, combine the milk, rice, water, apples, sugar, vanilla, and cinnamon stick.

2. Secure the lid and cook on high pressure for 12 minutes, then quick release the pressure and remove the lid. Press cancel.

3. In a small bowl, whisk the egg with ½ cup of the cooked rice pudding and return it to the pudding along with the half-and-half.

4. Select sauté and cook for 2 to 3 minutes, stirring the mixture well, to thicken the pudding.

5. Discard the cinnamon stick and serve warm.

INGREDIENT TIP: I recommend jasmine rice or long-grain Thai rice here.

Easy Frozen Berry Crisp

SERVES 6
PREP TIME: 5 MINUTES • COOK TIME: 12 MINUTES • TOTAL TIME: 40 MINUTES
PRESSURE RELEASE: NATURAL
UNDER AN HOUR, VEGETARIAN

Frozen berries are an ingredient I always keep in my freezer. This berry crisp is so easy, and you don't even need to thaw the berries. I always add lemon juice and zest when I make berry desserts, and the nutty oatmeal topping tastes out of this world! This dessert comes together easily and quickly.

12 ounces frozen berries (no need to thaw)

¼ cup granulated sugar

Grated zest of 1 lemon

3 tablespoons freshly squeezed lemon juice

¼ cup all-purpose flour

¼ cup rolled oats

¼ cup slivered almonds

1 tablespoon light brown sugar

½ teaspoon sea salt

3 tablespoons butter, cut into thin slices

1 cup water

1. In an ovenproof bowl or pan that fits in the inner pot, toss together the berries, granulated sugar, lemon zest, and lemon juice.

2. In a medium bowl, combine the flour, oats, almonds, brown sugar, and salt. Sprinkle the oatmeal topping over the frozen berries.

3. Place the butter slices on top of the oatmeal topping and cover the bowl with foil.

4. Pour the water into the pot and insert a trivet or a silicone sling (if you don't have a sling or a trivet with handles, fashion a foil sling and place it on the trivet). Place the covered bowl or pan on top.

5. Secure the lid and cook on high pressure for 12 minutes, then allow the pressure to naturally release. Press cancel.

6. Remove the lid and carefully lift out the bowl or pan using the handles of the trivet or sling.

7. If desired, uncover the bowl or pan and broil for 2 to 3 minutes in the oven for a crispier topping.

STORAGE: Refrigerate in a sealed container for up to 5 days.

INGREDIENT TIP: You can also use fresh berries in this recipe. Use 12 ounces and add ½ cup of water.

Chocolate Pudding

SERVES 6

PREP TIME: 5 MINUTES • COOK TIME: 20 MINUTES • TOTAL TIME: 35 MINUTES

PRESSURE RELEASE: QUICK

UNDER AN HOUR, VEGETARIAN

Once you start making homemade chocolate pudding in your electric pressure cooker, you won't go back to buying boxed pudding mix. This pudding recipe is foolproof and turns out rich and creamy every time. Add a little more cocoa powder for an extra chocolaty pudding.

1 large egg

⅓ cup sugar

3 tablespoons unsweetened cocoa powder

2 cups whole milk

1 tablespoon butter

1 tablespoon pure vanilla extract

1 tablespoon cornstarch

1 cup water

1. In a 7½-inch (or smaller) metal bowl, beat together the egg and sugar and whisk for about 30 seconds. Whisk in the cocoa until smooth, then whisk in the milk, butter, and vanilla. Whisk in the cornstarch until smooth, between 30 and 60 seconds.

2. Cover the bowl with aluminum foil.

3. Pour the water into the pot and insert a trivet or a silicone sling (if you don't have a sling or a trivet with handles, fashion a foil sling and place it on the trivet). Place the covered bowl on top.

4. Secure the lid and cook on high pressure for 20 minutes, then quick release the pressure and remove the lid.

5. Lift out the bowl using the trivet handles or sling. Once cooled, refrigerate the pudding to chill and set before serving.

Tapioca Pudding

SERVES 4
PREP TIME: 5 MINUTES • COOK TIME: 6 MINUTES • TOTAL TIME: 30 MINUTES
PRESSURE RELEASE: NATURAL
GLUTEN-FREE, UNDER AN HOUR, VEGETARIAN

When I was growing up, my mom would often make tapioca pudding for dessert. Usually, it was when we had an overabundance of milk in the house. I have always been partial to tapioca pudding, probably because of its texture. You can serve this pudding warm or cold, but I have always preferred it warm.

3 cups water

1 cup medium tapioca pearls

2 cups whole milk

½ cup sugar

1 large egg

1 tablespoon pure vanilla extract

½ teaspoon sea salt

1. In the inner pot, combine the water and tapioca pearls.

2. Secure the lid and cook on high pressure for 6 minutes, then allow the pressure to naturally release. Press cancel.

3. Remove the lid and stir in the milk, sugar, egg, vanilla, and salt while the tapioca is still piping hot.

4. You can serve this pudding warm or let chill in the refrigerator.

INGREDIENT TIP: I suggest Bob's Red Mill medium tapioca pearls for this recipe.

Ramekin Brownies

SERVES 4

PREP TIME: 5 MINUTES • COOK TIME: 7 MINUTES • TOTAL TIME: 30 MINUTES

PRESSURE RELEASE: NATURAL

UNDER AN HOUR, VEGETARIAN

When I first started making these personal-size brownies in my electric pressure cooker, I was trying to improve on the popular microwave mug brownies. I found the microwave mug version to be incredibly dry. The electric pressure cooker recipe tastes moist, delectable, fudgy, and chocolaty—the perfect quick treat to enjoy on a whim.

Nonstick cooking spray

½ cup all-purpose flour

6 tablespoons unsweetened cocoa powder

¼ cup sugar

½ teaspoon sea salt

4 tablespoons (½ stick) butter, melted

¼ cup whole milk

1 large egg

¼ cup chocolate chips

1 cup water

1. Mist each of 4 (2-inch) ramekins with cooking spray and set aside.

2. In a medium bowl, combine the flour, cocoa, sugar, and salt. Add the melted butter, milk, egg, and chocolate chips and mix well.

3. Divide the brownie batter among the ramekins (about ⅓ cup batter each). Cover each ramekin with foil.

4. Pour the water into the pot and insert a trivet or a silicone sling. Arrange the ramekins on the trivet or sling.

5. Secure the lid and cook on high pressure for 7 minutes. Allow the pressure to naturally release for 7 minutes, then quick release the remaining pressure and remove the lid. Press cancel.

6. Remove the trivet or sling from the pot. If your trivet does not have handles, use an oven mitt to carefully lift out the ramekins.

7. Remove the foil and serve the brownies in the ramekins while still warm.

STORAGE: Refrigerate in a sealed container for up to 5 days.

MEAL PLANNING TIP: These brownies make a delicious dessert for "at-home date night." I love serving them for dessert to follow my Garlic and Rosemary Lamb Chops (page 197).

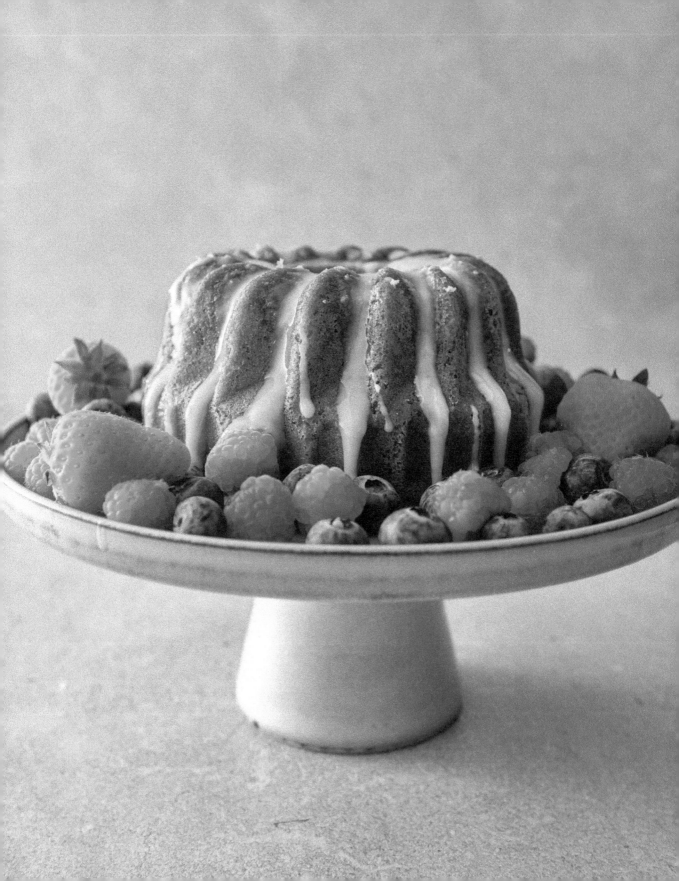

Vanilla Greek Yogurt Bundt Cake

SERVES 4 TO 6
PREP TIME: 10 MINUTES • COOK TIME: 35 MINUTES • TOTAL TIME: 1 HOUR
10 MINUTES
▶ **PRESSURE RELEASE:** NATURAL
VEGETARIAN, WORTH THE WAIT

Everyone should have a simple cake recipe that they can whip up on a whim and dress up for any occasion. This cake is just that. It is sweet, citrusy, and loaded with vanilla flavor. You can add chocolate, fruit, whipped cream, or glaze on top for delicious variations. The options are endless. When you make a cake in your electric pressure cooker, the cake will turn out perfectly fluffy in practically no time at all.

Nonstick cooking spray

1½ cups all-purpose flour

⅔ cup sugar

2 teaspoons baking powder

½ teaspoon baking soda

½ teaspoon sea salt

½ cup plain Greek yogurt, store-bought or homemade (page 228)

⅓ cup whole milk

4 tablespoons (½ stick) butter, at room temperature

1 large egg

1 tablespoon pure vanilla extract

Grated zest of 1 lemon

1 cup water

1. Mist a 7-inch Bundt pan with cooking spray.

2. In a medium bowl, combine the flour, sugar, baking powder, baking soda, and salt. Add the yogurt, milk, butter, egg, vanilla, and lemon zest and mix well.

3. Pour the water into the inner pot.

4. Pour the cake batter into the Bundt pan and cover it with foil. Place the pan onto a silicone sling or trivet with handles and lower the cake into the pot. (If you don't have a sling or a trivet with handles, fashion a foil sling and use it to lower the pan onto a regular trivet in the pot.)

5. Secure the lid and cook on high pressure for 35 minutes, then allow the pressure to naturally release. Press cancel and remove the lid.

▶
CONTINUED

6. Carefully lift out the pan using the handles of the trivet or sling. Remove the foil and let the cake cool before unmolding.

7. Cut the cake into slices and serve.

STORAGE: Refrigerate in a sealed container for up to 5 days.

MENU PLANNING TIP: I love topping this cake with fresh berries!

Pie Filling Dump Cake

SERVES 6
PREP TIME: 5 MINUTES • COOK TIME: 8 MINUTES • TOTAL TIME: 25 MINUTES
PRESSURE RELEASE: QUICK
UNDER 30 MINUTES, VEGETARIAN

Creating a dump cake in your electric pressure cooker might be the easiest dessert you can make. You literally "dump" the ingredients into the pot; it cooks up fast and will please everyone. You can use any pie filling you like, such as cherry, apple, blueberry, or strawberry. All are equally delicious, but peach is my favorite. The ice cream and whipped cream for topping the cake are listed as optional here, but I personally consider them a must.

1¼ cups all-purpose flour

1 cup sugar

1 teaspoon baking powder

½ teaspoon sea salt

½ cup water

1 (15-ounce) can pie filling

4 tablespoons (½ stick) butter, cut into slices

Vanilla ice cream, for serving (optional)

Whipped cream, for serving (optional)

1. In a medium bowl, mix together the flour, sugar, baking powder, and salt.

2. Pour the water into the pressure cooker pot. Pour the pie filling on top of the water and do not mix. Add the flour mixture on top of the pie filling and do not mix.

3. Dot the top with the butter.

4. Secure the lid and cook on high pressure for 8 minutes, then quick release the pressure and remove the lid. Press cancel.

5. Serve heaping spoonfuls of cake in dessert bowls. If desired, top with ice cream or whipped cream.

STORAGE: Refrigerate in a sealed container for up to 5 days.

RECIPE TOOLBOX: If you want to simplify this, you can use a boxed cake mix instead of the cake ingredients here. Use 1 (15-ounce) box of cake mix and omit the flour, sugar, baking powder, and salt.

9 Staples

Vegetable Broth

MAKES ABOUT 7 CUPS
PREP TIME: 10 MINUTES • COOK TIME: 20 MINUTES • TOTAL TIME: 50 MINUTES
PRESSURE RELEASE: NATURAL
DAIRY-FREE, ESSENTIAL RECIPE, GLUTEN-FREE, UNDER AN HOUR, VEGAN

Making vegetable broth in your electric pressure cooker is so simple that you won't need to buy it anymore. All you need is a few ingredients and spices to make a delicious-tasting broth. I make this when I'm making a vegetarian soup, but I also make a batch and freeze it to use in other recipes.

8 cups water

1½ cups chopped celery

3 carrots, cut into chunks

1 onion, chopped

3 garlic cloves

1 teaspoon herbes de Provence

1 bay leaf

1. In the inner pot, combine the water, celery, carrots, onion, garlic, herbes de Provence, and bay leaf.

2. Secure the lid and cook on high pressure for 20 minutes, then allow the pressure to naturally release. Press cancel and remove the lid.

3. Set a sieve over a large bowl. Strain the vegetable broth into the bowl (discard the veggie scraps).

4. Use immediately or store.

STORAGE: Refrigerate in a sealed container for up to 5 days or freeze for up to 6 months.

Chicken Stock

MAKES ABOUT 7 CUPS
PREP TIME: 10 MINUTES • COOK TIME: 20 MINUTES • TOTAL TIME: 50 MINUTES
PRESSURE RELEASE: NATURAL
DAIRY-FREE, GLUTEN-FREE, UNDER AN HOUR

I like to prepare chicken stock at night after a chicken dinner. I think it's easier to "deal with the bones" right away. I used to leave chicken stock simmering in my slow cooker overnight, but making it in the electric pressure cooker is much easier and takes a fraction of the time. Many recipes in this book call for chicken stock, so it is a great ingredient to have handy.

8 cups water

1 whole chicken carcass or 2 pounds leftover chicken bones

½ onion, chopped

1 garlic clove

1 tablespoon freshly squeezed lemon juice

1 teaspoon dried rosemary

1 bay leaf

1. In the inner pot, combine the water, chicken bones, onion, garlic, lemon juice, rosemary, and bay leaf.

2. Secure the lid and cook on high pressure for 20 minutes, then allow the pressure to naturally release. Press cancel and remove the lid.

3. Set a sieve over a large bowl. Strain the chicken stock into the bowl (discard the chicken bones and vegetables). Skim the fat off the chicken stock once it has cooled.

4. Use immediately or store.

STORAGE: Refrigerate in a sealed container for up to 5 days or freeze for up to 6 months.

Beef Stock

MAKES ABOUT 7 CUPS
PREP TIME: 10 MINUTES • COOK TIME: 30 MINUTES • TOTAL TIME: 50 MINUTES
PRESSURE RELEASE: NATURAL
DAIRY-FREE, GLUTEN-FREE, UNDER AN HOUR

One thing I love about my electric pressure cooker is creating "round-two" recipes from leftovers. When I buy a nice piece of bone-in beef, I always turn it into stock afterward. Beef stock is full of nutrients and can be used in a variety of delicious recipes. If you don't have any leftover beef bones handy, you can also purchase bones from your butcher.

4 pounds large beef bones with marrow or leftover short ribs, pot roast bones, or steak bones

8 cups water

1 onion, quartered

2 carrots, cut into 1-inch chunks

1 celery stalk, cut into 2-inch chunks

2 garlic cloves, peeled

1 teaspoon dried rosemary

1. In the inner pot, combine the beef bones, water, onion, carrots, celery, garlic, and rosemary.

2. Secure the lid and cook on high pressure for 30 minutes, then allow the pressure to naturally release. Press cancel and remove the lid.

3. Set a sieve over a large bowl. Strain the beef stock into the bowl (discard the bones and vegetables). Skim the fat off the stock once it has cooled.

4. Use immediately or store.

STORAGE: Refrigerate in a sealed container for up to 5 days or freeze for up to 6 months.

Sweet and Smoky Barbecue Sauce

MAKES 2 CUPS
PREP TIME: 10 MINUTES • COOK TIME: 21 MINUTES • TOTAL TIME: 30 MINUTES
PRESSURE RELEASE: QUICK
DAIRY-FREE, GLUTEN-FREE, UNDER AN HOUR, VEGETARIAN

There is nothing quite like using homemade high-quality barbecue sauce in your kitchen. This sauce happens to be a favorite in my house. It is easy to make and tastes delicious with a variety of different meals.

1 tablespoon vegetable oil

1 small onion, finely chopped

1 (15-ounce) can tomato sauce

1 cup water

½ cup distilled white vinegar

⅓ cup packed light brown sugar

2 garlic cloves, minced

2 teaspoons liquid smoke

1 teaspoon chili powder

1 teaspoon ground cumin

1. Select sauté and let the pot heat up for 2 minutes.

2. Add the oil and onion and sauté for 2 to 3 minutes, or until the onion is translucent.

3. Add the tomato sauce, water, vinegar, brown sugar, garlic, liquid smoke, chili powder, and cumin.

4. Secure the lid and cook on high pressure for 8 minutes, then quick release the pressure and remove the lid.

5. Select sauté and cook, stirring occasionally, for 10 minutes, or until the barbecue sauce reduces by half.

6. Let the barbecue sauce cool before serving or storing.

STORAGE: Refrigerate in a sealed container for up to 2 weeks.

MENU PLANNING TIP: Use this sweet and smoky barbecue sauce in Smoky Barbecue Ribs (page 177), Smoky Barbecue Sticky Chicken Wings (page 147), and Large-Batch Smoky Barbecue Pork Chop Sandwiches (page 172).

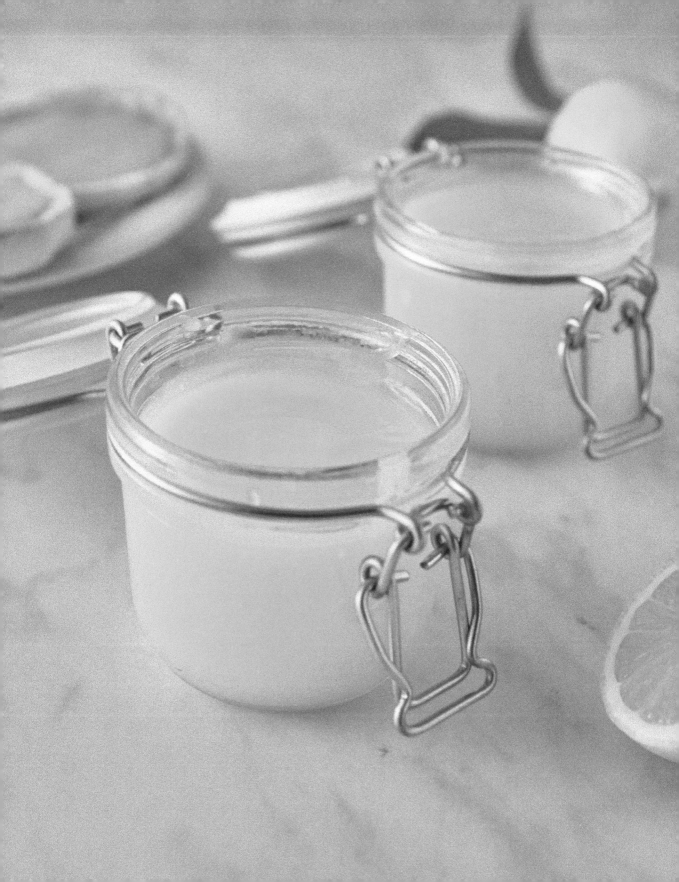

Lemon Curd

MAKES 2 CUPS
PREP TIME: 10 MINUTES • COOK TIME: 10 MINUTES • TOTAL TIME: 40 MINUTES
PRESSURE RELEASE: NATURAL
GLUTEN-FREE, UNDER AN HOUR, VEGETARIAN

I fell in love with lemon curd when all the women in my family started attending "high tea" every Christmas in Chicagoland. The lemon curd was always served with our scones. When I learned that lemon curd could be made quickly in an electric pressure cooker, I instantly tried it. My family loves topping yogurt with this luscious curd or spreading it on muffins and toast.

¾ cup sugar

5 tablespoons butter, at room temperature

Grated zest of 1 lemon

1 cup freshly squeezed lemon juice

3 large eggs

2 large egg yolks

1 cup water

1. In a medium bowl, with a hand mixer, blend the sugar, butter, and lemon zest together.

2. Beat in the lemon juice, whole eggs, and egg yolks and mix well. The mixture won't be completely smooth.

3. Transfer the mixture to a 7-inch glass bowl and cover it with foil.

4. Pour the water into the pot and place the bowl onto a silicone sling or trivet with handles and lower the bowl into the pot. (If you don't have a sling or a trivet with handles, fashion a foil sling and use it to lower the bowl onto a regular trivet in the pot.)

5. Secure the lid and cook on high pressure for 10 minutes, then allow the pressure to naturally release for at least 10 minutes (as the curd will continue cooking during this time). Press cancel and remove the lid.

6. Carefully lift out the bowl using the handles of the trivet or sling.

7. Cool in the refrigerator before serving.

STORAGE: Refrigerate in a sealed container for up to 2 weeks.

Yogurt

MAKES 7 CUPS

PREP TIME: 10 MINUTES • COOK TIME: 10 HOURS • TOTAL TIME: 10 HOURS

GLUTEN-FREE, VEGETARIAN, WORTH THE WAIT

My sugar palate has changed over the years, making most store-bought yogurts too sweet for my taste. I enjoy making homemade yogurt in my electric pressure cooker because I can control the sweetness of the toppings I choose to add. This is an all-day process, but it is hands-off, and the yogurt is perfectly creamy and rich. Once you try it, you will always make it this way.

8 cups whole milk

2 tablespoons plain yogurt with active cultures

1. Pour the milk into the inner pot. Secure the lid and leave the pressure release valve set to "venting."

2. Select the "yogurt" mode and press the button two times. The display on the control panel should say "boil."

3. Once the boiling process is completed, about 30 minutes, open the lid and check the milk's temperature. It needs to reach 180°F. Let the milk cool until it reaches 115°F, about 1 hour.

4. Remove the thin film on top of the milk with a spoon, whisk in the yogurt with active cultures, cover, and secure the lid. Again leave the pressure release valve set to "venting."

5. Press the "yogurt" button (just once). The display on the control panel should read "8.00." The cooking process for yogurt is 8 hours. Don't open the pressure cooker lid until the 8 hours are completed. At the end of this time, the yogurt should be creamy and thick.

6. Store it in containers and refrigerate overnight.

7. For a thicker, Greek-style yogurt: Spoon the yogurt into a sieve lined with dampened cheesecloth and set the sieve over a bowl. Let the yogurt drain off liquid until it reaches the consistency you prefer. (Discard the whey.)

STORAGE: Refrigerate in a sealed container for up to 2 weeks.

INGREDIENT TIP: Most plain store-bought yogurt will work, but make sure it has active cultures. Check the label for the ingredients *Lactobacillus bulgaricus* or *Streptococcus thermophilus*.

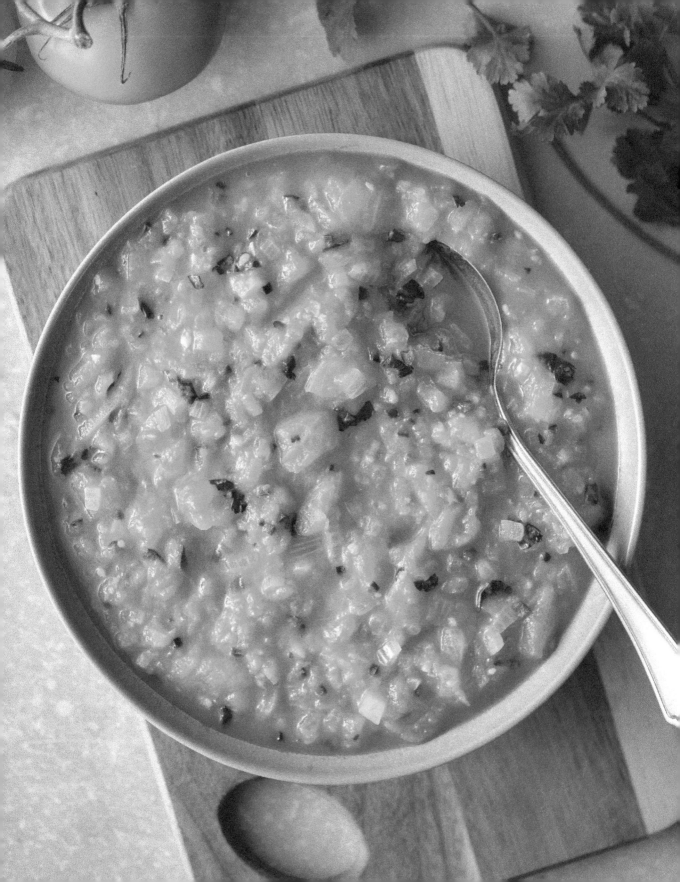

Garden Salsa

MAKES ABOUT 4 CUPS
PREP TIME: 5 MINUTES • COOK TIME: 5 MINUTES • TOTAL TIME: 30 MINUTES
PRESSURE RELEASE: NATURAL
DAIRY-FREE, GLUTEN-FREE, UNDER AN HOUR, VEGAN

There is something about homemade freshly blended salsa that jarred salsa can never match. Every summer we grow tomatoes and jalapeño peppers in our garden, and toward the end of the season we make homemade salsa. If you don't have fresh garden tomatoes, you can use a can of high-quality tomatoes for this recipe.

15 tomatoes, halved
or 1 (35-ounce) can
whole tomatoes

1 large onion, finely chopped

2 jalapeño peppers, seeded
and finely chopped

4 garlic cloves, minced

½ cup chopped
fresh cilantro

1 teaspoon sea salt

1. In the inner pot, combine the tomatoes, onion, jalapeños, garlic, cilantro, and salt.

2. Secure the lid and cook on high pressure for 5 minutes, then allow the pressure to naturally release. Press cancel.

3. Remove the lid. Pulse with an immersion blender (or transfer to a stand blender) so that it is combined but still chunky.

4. Use immediately or store.

STORAGE: Refrigerate in a sealed container for up to 5 days or freeze for up to 2 months.

INGREDIENT TIP: Increase or reduce the amount of jalapeño peppers in this recipe to achieve your desired heat level.

Marinara Sauce

MAKES 3 CUPS
PREP TIME: 15 MINUTES • COOK TIME: 12 MINUTES • TOTAL TIME: 40 MINUTES
PRESSURE RELEASE: NATURAL
DAIRY-FREE, GLUTEN-FREE, UNDER AN HOUR, VEGAN

Marinara sauce was one of the first recipes that I "made my own." In college, I started experimenting with homemade marinara sauce recipes when I cooked for my roommates. In my opinion, the secret ingredient in marinara sauce is carrots. Carrots cut down on the acidity of the tomatoes and act as a natural sweetener. Making your own homemade marinara sauce in the electric pressure cooker not only saves time, but it is much less messy: You don't need to worry about simmering sauce splattering all over your stovetop (and you).

⅓ cup olive oil

5 shallots, chopped

6 garlic cloves, minced

10 to 12 tomatoes, halved, or 1 (28-ounce) can whole tomatoes

4 carrots, sliced

1 cup water

2 tablespoons Italian seasoning

Sea salt

Freshly ground black pepper

1. Select sauté and let the pot heat up for 2 minutes.

2. Add the olive oil, shallots, and garlic and sauté for about 2 minutes, or until the shallots are translucent.

3. Add the tomatoes, carrots, water, and Italian seasoning.

4. Secure the lid and cook on high pressure for 10 minutes, then allow the pressure to naturally release. Press cancel.

5. Remove the lid. Puree with an immersion blender (or transfer to a stand blender and puree) until smooth. Taste and season with salt and pepper as needed.

6. Use or store for later.

STORAGE: Refrigerate in a sealed container for up to 5 days or freeze for up to 2 months.

MENU PLANNING TIP: This Marinara Sauce tastes wonderful when used to make Gnocchi Lasagna (page 110).

Applesauce

MAKES 5 CUPS
PREP TIME: 15 MINUTES • COOK TIME: 10 MINUTES • TOTAL TIME: 1 HOUR
5 MINUTES
PRESSURE RELEASE: QUICK
DAIRY-FREE, GLUTEN-FREE, WORTH THE WAIT, VEGAN

My family enjoys apple picking almost every year. We always pick more apples than we can carry, leaving us with no choice but to make a large batch of delicious cinnamon applesauce. This recipe calls for 10 red apples and 2 green apples to give the sauce the perfect amount of tartness. For years, I made my applesauce in the slow cooker, but now I've learned how to speed up the process using the electric pressure cooker instead.

10 red apples, peeled, cored, and cut into 1-inch chunks

2 Granny Smith apples, peeled, cored, and cut into 1-inch chunks

½ cup packed light brown sugar

¼ cup freshly squeezed lemon juice

¼ cup water

2 cinnamon sticks or 2 teaspoons ground cinnamon

1. In the inner pot, combine the red and Granny Smith apples, brown sugar, lemon juice, water, and cinnamon sticks.

2. Secure the lid and cook on high pressure for 10 minutes, then quick release the pressure and remove the lid. Press cancel.

3. If you want your applesauce smooth, blend it with an immersion blender.

4. Eat immediately or store.

STORAGE: Refrigerate in a sealed container for up to 1 week.

MENU PLANNING TIP: This applesauce shines as an ingredient in the Cinnamon Applesauce Pork Chops (page 171).

Balsamic Ketchup

MAKES 1½ CUPS
PREP TIME: 15 MINUTES • COOK TIME: 23 MINUTES • TOTAL TIME: 35 MINUTES
PRESSURE RELEASE: QUICK
DAIRY-FREE, GLUTEN-FREE, UNDER AN HOUR, VEGAN

Ketchup is probably the most consumed condiment in my house. My kids like adding it to many of the foods we serve. Once we discovered balsamic-spiked ketchup, we never turned back. Making homemade ketchup is much less expensive than the store-bought version, and it tastes so much better, too!

1 (15-ounce) can
tomato sauce

1 cup water

½ cup balsamic vinegar

¼ cup sugar

1 tablespoon onion powder

1 teaspoon garlic powder

1 teaspoon sea salt

1. In the inner pot, combine the tomato sauce, water, vinegar, sugar, onion powder, garlic powder, and salt.

2. Secure the lid and cook on high pressure for 8 minutes, then quick release the pressure and remove the lid. Press cancel.

3. Select sauté and cook, stirring occasionally, for about 15 minutes to thicken and reduce the ketchup.

4. Let the ketchup cool before serving or storing.

STORAGE: Refrigerate in an airtight container for up to 2 weeks.

MENU PLANNING TIP: This balsamic ketchup tastes excellent with the Salted Baby Potatoes (page 60).

Caramelized Shallots

MAKES 1 CUP
PREP TIME: 10 MINUTES • COOK TIME: 25 MINUTES • TOTAL TIME: 50 MINUTES
PRESSURE RELEASE: QUICK
DAIRY-FREE, GLUTEN-FREE, UNDER AN HOUR, VEGAN

Shallots are one of my favorite ingredients to keep handy. They are sweeter than onions and have tons of garlicky flavor, as well. I like to keep these caramelized shallots in ice cube trays in my freezer so that I can pop one out when I need it for a quick recipe. I spent a lot of time caramelizing shallots over the stove, but the electric pressure cooker is an easy hands-off way to achieve the same results.

5 to 6 tablespoons olive oil, divided

2 pounds shallots, peeled and cut into ½-inch slices

¼ cup water

1. Pour 5 tablespoons of olive oil into the inner pot and add the shallots. Toss the shallots with the oil to thoroughly coat. Add the water.

2. Secure the lid and cook on high pressure for 20 minutes, then quick release the pressure and remove the lid. Press cancel.

3. Select sauté and cook the shallots for 5 more minutes, or until they are browned to your liking. You may want to add the remaining 1 tablespoon of olive oil at this time.

4. Use immediately or freeze for up to 3 months.

INGREDIENT TIP: This cooking method will also work for onions. Since onions are larger, after pressure-cooking, you will want to sauté them for a few minutes longer.

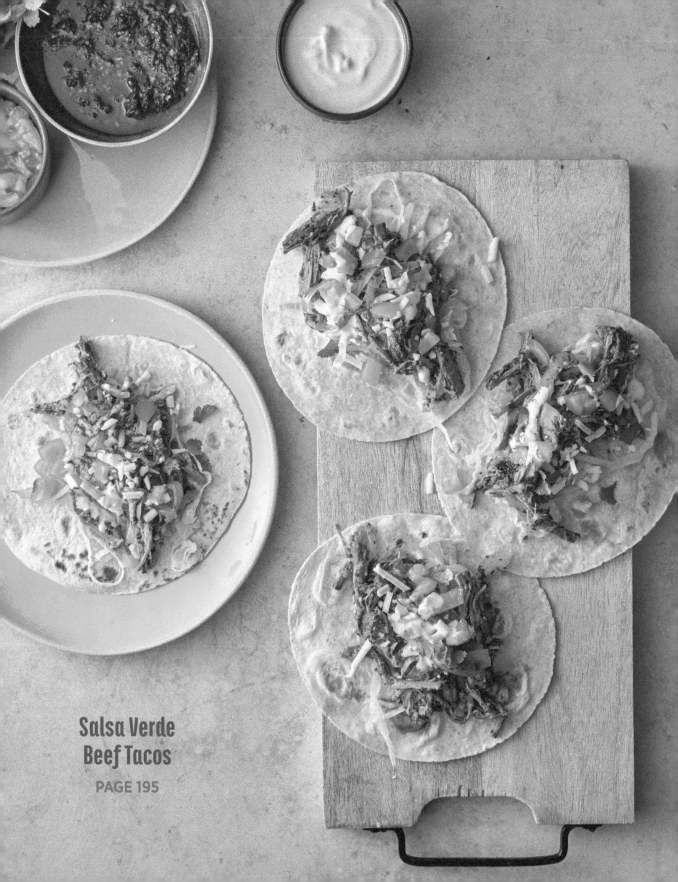

Salsa Verde
Beef Tacos

PAGE 195

Pressure-Cooking Time Charts

These charts provide approximate cooking times for a variety of foods. Keep in mind that these times are for the foods partially submerged in water or broth or steamed and for the foods cooked by themselves in the pot. The cooking times for the same foods when they are part of a recipe may differ because of additional ingredients or cooking liquids or a different release method than the one listed here. For any foods labeled "natural" release, allow at least 10 minutes of natural pressure release before quick releasing any remaining pressure.

BEANS AND LEGUMES

Unless otherwise noted, the bean cooking times are for dried beans that have been soaked for 8 to 24 hours in salted water. But you can cook *unsoaked* beans in the pressure cooker; you'll just need to increase the cooking time—often up to 1 hour more.

When cooking beans, if you have a pound or more, it's best to use low pressure and increase the cooking time by a minute or two. Cooking larger amounts at high pressure increases the chance of foaming. If you have less than a pound, high pressure is fine. A little oil in the cooking liquid will reduce foaming. Where two times are listed, the shorter time is for high pressure and the longer time is for low pressure.

	LIQUID PER 1 CUP BEANS (ABOUT 3 OUNCES)	MINUTES UNDER PRESSURE	PRESSURE LEVEL	RELEASE
BEANS, BLACK	2 cups	8 to 9	High / Low	Natural
BEANS, CANNELLINI	2 cups	5 to 7	High / Low	Natural
BEANS, KIDNEY	2 cups	5 to 7	High / Low	Natural
BEANS, PINTO	2 cups	8 to 10	High / Low	Natural
BLACK-EYED PEAS	2 cups	5	High	Natural for 8 minutes, then quick
CHICKPEAS (GARBANZO BEANS)	2 cups	4	High	Natural for 3 minutes, then quick
LENTILS, BROWN (UNSOAKED)	2¼ cups	20	High	Natural for 10 minutes, then quick
LENTILS, RED (UNSOAKED)	3 cups	10	High	Natural for 5 minutes, then quick
LIMA BEANS	2 cups	4 to 5	High / Low	Natural for 5 minutes, then quick
SOYBEANS, GREEN, FRESH (EDAMAME)	1 cup	1	High	Quick
SOYBEANS, DRIED	2 cups	12 to 14	High / Low	Natural
SPLIT PEAS (UNSOAKED)	3 cups	5 (firm peas) to 8 (soft peas)	High	Natural

GRAINS

To prevent foaming, it's best to include a small amount of butter or oil with the cooking liquid for these grains or to rinse them thoroughly before cooking.

	LIQUID PER 1 CUP GRAIN	MINUTES UNDER PRESSURE	PRESSURE LEVEL	RELEASE
BARLEY, PEARL	2½ cups	20	High	Natural for 10 minutes, then quick
BUCKWHEAT	1¾ cups	2 to 4	High	Natural
FARRO, PEARLED	2 cups	6 to 8	High	Natural
FARRO, WHOLE GRAIN	3 cups	22 to 24	High	Natural
OATS, ROLLED	3 cups	3 to 4	High	Quick
OATS, STEEL-CUT	3 cups	10	High	Natural for 10 minutes, then quick
QUINOA	1 cup	2	High	Natural for 12 minutes, then quick
RICE, ARBORIO (FOR RISOTTO)	3 to 4 cups	6 to 8	High	Quick
RICE, BROWN, LONG-GRAIN	1 cup	22	High	Natural for 10 minutes, then quick
RICE, BROWN, MEDIUM-GRAIN	1 cup	12	High	Natural
RICE, WHITE, LONG-GRAIN	1 cup	3	High	Natural
WHEAT BERRIES	2 cups	30	High	Natural for 10 minutes, then quick
WILD RICE	1¼ cups	22 to 24	High	Natural

MEATS

Except as noted, these times are for braised meats—that is, meats that are seared first and then pressure-cooked partially submerged in liquid.

	MINUTES UNDER PRESSURE	PRESSURE LEVEL	RELEASE
BEEF, BONE-IN SHORT RIBS	40	High	Natural
BEEF, SHOULDER (CHUCK) ROAST (2 POUNDS)	35 to 45	High	Natural
BEEF, SHOULDER (CHUCK), 2-INCH CHUNKS	20	High	Natural for 10 minutes, then quick
BEEF, FLATIRON STEAK, CUT INTO ½-INCH STRIPS	6	Low	Quick
BEEF, SIRLOIN STEAK, CUT INTO ½-INCH STRIPS	3	Low	Quick
LAMB, SHANKS	40	High	Natural
LAMB, SHOULDER, 2-INCH CHUNKS	35	High	Natural
PORK, BACK RIBS (STEAMED)	25 (steamed)	High	Quick
PORK, SHOULDER, 2-INCH CHUNKS	20	High	Quick
PORK, SHOULDER ROAST (2 POUNDS)	25	High	Natural
PORK, SMOKED SAUSAGE, ½-INCH SLICES	5 to 10	High	Quick
PORK, SPARE RIBS (STEAMED)	20 (steamed)	High	Quick
PORK, TENDERLOIN	4	Low	Quick

POULTRY

Except as noted, these times are for braised poultry—that is, partially submerged in liquid during cooking.

	MINUTES UNDER PRESSURE	PRESSURE LEVEL	RELEASE
CHICKEN BREAST, BONE-IN (STEAMED)	8	Low	Natural for 5 minutes, then quick
CHICKEN BREAST, BONELESS (STEAMED)	5	Low	Natural for 8 minutes, then quick
CHICKEN THIGH, BONE-IN	10 to 14	High	Natural for 10 minutes, then quick
CHICKEN THIGH, BONELESS	6 to 8	High	Natural for 10 minutes, then quick
CHICKEN THIGH, BONELESS, 1- TO 2-INCH PIECES	5 to 6	High	Quick
CHICKEN, WHOLE (SEARED ON ALL SIDES)	12 to 14	Low	Natural for 8 minutes, then quick
DUCK QUARTERS, BONE-IN	35	High	Quick
TURKEY BREAST, TENDERLOIN (12 OUNCES) (STEAMED)	5	Low	Natural for 8 minutes, then quick
TURKEY THIGH, BONE-IN	30	High	Natural

FISH AND SEAFOOD

All times are for steamed fish and shellfish.

	MINUTES UNDER PRESSURE	PRESSURE LEVEL	RELEASE
CLAMS	2	High	Quick
HALIBUT, FRESH (1 INCH THICK)	3	High	Quick
MUSSELS	1	High	Quick
SALMON, FRESH (1 INCH THICK)	5	Low	Quick
TILAPIA OR COD, FRESH	1	Low	Quick
TILAPIA OR COD, FROZEN	3	Low	Quick
LARGE SHRIMP, FROZEN	1	Low	Quick

VEGETABLES

The cooking method for all the following vegetables is steaming; if the vegetables are cooked in liquid, the times may vary. Green vegetables will be tender-crisp; root vegetables will be soft.

	PREP	MINUTES UNDER PRESSURE	PRESSURE LEVEL	RELEASE
ACORN SQUASH	Halved	9	High	Quick
ARTICHOKES, LARGE	Whole	15	High	Quick
BEETS	Quartered if large, halved if small	9	High	Natural
BROCCOLI	Cut into florets	1	Low	Quick
BRUSSELS SPROUTS	Halved	2	High	Quick
BUTTERNUT SQUASH	Peeled, cut into ½-inch chunks	8	High	Quick
CABBAGE	Sliced	3 to 4	High	Quick
CARROTS	½- to 1-inch slices	2	High	Quick
CAULIFLOWER	Whole	6	High	Quick
CAULIFLOWER	Cut into florets	0 to 1	Low	Quick
GREEN BEANS	Cut in half or thirds	3	Low	Quick
POTATOES, LARGE RUSSET (FOR MASHING)	Quartered	8	High	Natural for 8 minutes, then quick
POTATOES, RED	Whole if less than 1½ inches across, halved if larger	4	High	Quick
SPAGHETTI SQUASH	Halved lengthwise	7	High	Quick
SWEET POTATOES	Halved lengthwise	8	High	Natural

Measurement Conversions

	US STANDARD	US STANDARD (OUNCES)	METRIC (APPROXIMATE)
VOLUME EQUIVALENTS (LIQUID)	2 TABLESPOONS	1 FL. OZ.	30 ML
	¼ CUP	2 FL. OZ.	60 ML
	½ CUP	4 FL. OZ.	120 ML
	1 CUP	8 FL. OZ.	240 ML
	1½ CUPS	12 FL. OZ.	355 ML
	2 CUPS OR 1 PINT	16 FL. OZ.	475 ML
	4 CUPS OR 1 QUART	32 FL. OZ.	1 L
	1 GALLON	128 FL. OZ.	4 L
VOLUME EQUIVALENTS (DRY)	⅛ TEASPOON		0.5 ML
	¼ TEASPOON		1 ML
	½ TEASPOON		2 ML
	¾ TEASPOON		4 ML
	1 TEASPOON		5 ML
	1 TABLESPOON		15 ML
	¼ CUP		59 ML
	⅓ CUP		79 ML
	½ CUP		118 ML
	⅔ CUP		156 ML
	¾ CUP		177 ML
	1 CUP		235 ML
	2 CUPS OR 1 PINT		475 ML
	3 CUPS		700 ML
	4 CUPS OR 1 QUART		1 L
	½ GALLON		2 L
	1 GALLON		4 L
WEIGHT EQUIVALENTS	½ OUNCE		15 G
	1 OUNCE		30 G
	2 OUNCES		60 G
	4 OUNCES		115 G
	8 OUNCES		225 G
	12 OUNCES		340 G
	16 OUNCES OR 1 POUND		455 G

	FAHRENHEIT (F)	CELSIUS (C) (APPROXIMATE)
OVEN TEMPERATURES	250°F	120°C
	300°F	150°C
	325°F	180°C
	375°F	190°C
	400°F	200°C
	425°F	220°C
	450°F	230°C

Resources

Amazon

Amazon.com

If there is ever a food item or product that I can't find here in Iowa, I like to search for it on Amazon. I enjoy looking for unique sauces, spice mixes, and items our stores don't have. I also buy cookbooks, pressure cooker accessories, cutting boards, and other utensils from Amazon. I even have an online store where I share my favorite products: In Google, just search for "Make the Best of Everything's Amazon page" to find it.

Make the Best of Everything

MaketTheBestOfEverything.com

My website is full of family-friendly recipes, including over 70 more electric pressure cooker recipes for you to check out.

The Spruce Eats

TheSpruceEats.com

The Spruce Eats is a food website that I enjoy. I especially love learning about the history of different ingredients and getting information on how to cook different cuisines. I also enjoy reading about the basics of a new-to-me ingredient before I try to cook with it.

Walmart

Walmart.com

I am a busy working mom of three kids. Ordering my groceries online saves me loads of time. Walmart.com is the most user-friendly website for ordering groceries for both pick-up and delivery. I forget ingredients less often when I shop for them online while I meal plan. Knowing what items are available in my area helps me plan out meals, plus I often develop new recipes based on the food products available at my local store.

Williams-Sonoma

WilliamsSonoma.com

Williams-Sonoma is my go-to source for kitchen gear that is sure to last. They have a large variety of electric pressure cookers, high-quality utensils, and cookbooks. I also love their starter sauces and their mixes. I enjoy shopping at Williams-Sonoma for gifts for family and friends.

Index

Acknowledgments

I want to thank the following people:

My mom and dad, for introducing me to a world of good food and unconditional love. I hit the jackpot in the parent department, and you taught me that I needed to find what I loved to do and work hard at it.

My husband, Greg, for being my best friend, always challenging me intellectually, and making my life exciting and wonderful. You stepped up your dad-game on nights and weekends so that I could get this book finished. Your support means the world to me and quarantining with you made me realize how much I love spending my life with you.

My three sons, Evan, Jack, and William. My three mini best friends. Every recipe has to be approved by you guys before it hits the press, and I can always count on your honesty. You three were great sports during this whole process. Eating four side dishes for dinner, suffering through lots of hot soup in the sweltering July heat, and taste-testing endless cheesecakes. Watching the three of you grow up is among life's greatest joys.

My Squad: Kurt, Brad, Celia, Sandra, Bridget, Alexis, Karen, Amy, and Maureen. Your support means everything to me. 24-hours-a-day texts; your efforts to help me test recipes; advice on food, life, kids, and quarantine; sending jokes and GIFs; and understanding my sarcasm—it has all meant the world. I am grateful to you.

Thank you to Callisto Media for reaching out to me and giving me this platform. I am blessed to receive this excellent opportunity.

About the Author

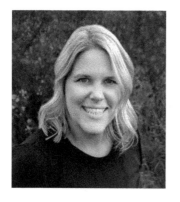

Kristen Greazel is a freelance recipe developer, food writer, photographer, and mother of three, born and raised in Chicagoland, now based in Iowa. She founded a popular recipe website, Make the Best of Everything (MakeTheBestOfEverything.com) where she shares easy and creative recipe tutorials, including many electric pressure cooker recipes. Her website and social media content reaches millions each year. When she isn't cooking, writing, or eating, she loves to travel, hike, explore, read, listen to podcasts, and spend time with family and friends. You can find Kristen on Instagram at @Kristen_MakeTheBest.

CPSIA information can be obtained
at www.ICGtesting.com
Printed in the USA
LVHW070723180721
692907LV00011B/23

9 781638 788126